The BEEF LOVER'S GUIDE
TO WEIGHT CONTROL AND LOWER CHOLESTEROL

The BEEF LOVER'S GUIDE
TO WEIGHT CONTROL AND LOWER CHOLESTEROL

by
Chriss McNaught

Illustrated by
Jerry Palen

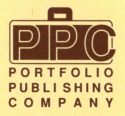

PORTFOLIO PUBLISHING COMPANY

P.O. Box 7802   The Woodlands, Texas 77387

Every effort has been made to trace the ownership of copyrighted materials and to secure permission from copyright holders. The recipes in this book come from the author's files which have been collected over a period of many years and the origination of many is therefore impossible to trace. In the event of any question arising as to the use of any material, we will be pleased to make the necessary corrections in future printings.

The information in this book reflects the author's experience and is not intended as medical advice. Any questions or concerns should be directed to your own physician.

Library of Congress Cataloging-in-Publication Data

The Beef Lover's Guide
to Weight Control and Lower Cholesterol

I. McNaught, Chriss, 1943-; illustrated by Jerry Palen
First Edition
p. 256 cm.

ISBN 0-943255-27-9 : $24.95
1. Reducing diets— Recipes. 2. Low-cholesterol diet— Recipes.
3. Cookery (Beef)
RM222.2.M437 1989
613.2'6— dc20

Copyright © 1989 by The Portfolio Publishing Company, The Wood-lands, Texas. All rights reserved. This books, or parts thereof, may not be reproduced in any form without express permission of the copyright holder.

ISBN 0-943255-27-9

Library of Congress Catalogue Number 89-25593

Printed in The United States of America
First Edition

Before beginning this or any other medical or dietary management regimen, please consult your physician to be sure that it is appropriate for you.

*This book is dedicated to my husband Ross,
for whom the recipes were originally developed and prepared.
By obligingly losing weight and lowering his cholesterol,
he proved that my theory really will work.*

*I would also like to thank my children and
my friends who have all been so supportive and
encouraging since I began this project.*

*Thanks to Arlene and Trisha for all their help, to Sandy for keeping
my life organized, to Ree Zaphiropoulos for sharing her philosophy
about salads, to Scott and Geraldine Haycock for generously
sharing the "Merlybird," and
to Met and Lana Johnson and Bill and Phyllis Callis
for all their extra efforts on my behalf.*

*And special thanks to Dixie Gregerson for her
endless faith in me.*

Table of Contents

Foreword   ix
 Enrique Alfaro, M.D.

Introduction   xiv
 Chriss McNaught

Jerry Palen, Illustrator   xviii

**A Note about the
  Dietary Analyses of the Recipes**   xix

Begin a New Lifestyle

Develop a Philosophy   3

The American Heart Association Guidelines   5

Weight Management   6

Desirable Weight Chart   10

Exercise   13

Energy Intake Chart   15

Calorie Expenditures   17

Get the Facts

Facts About	
Heart Disease	**23**
Fat	**26**
Cholesterol	**33**
Salt	**39**
Fiber	**43**
Adapting Your Own Recipes	**45**
The Daily Diet Menu Plan	**46**
Corraling Those Beef Facts	**47**

Beef, Wonderful Beef

*Individual contents are given at the beginning of each section
and in the index at the end of the Guide.*

Preparating and Serving Beef	**53**
Cooking Beef	**54**
Special Microwave Tricks	**61**
Carving Beef	**64**
The Salad: Beef's Perfect Complement	**65**
The Salad Philosophy	**66**
Ree Zaphiropoulos	
Beef Salads	**73**

Beef Soups	85
Beef Stir-Fry	95
Beef Burgers & Sandwiches	103
Beef Marinades	113
Beef Main Entrees	119

Entertaining with Beef

Menus for Four	151
Menus for Six	166
Menus for Eight	183
Party Menus	207
Index	231

Foreword

The American public is becoming increasingly concerned about cholesterol, fats, sugar, sodium, and additives in their diets. In our search for eternal youth, we diet and exercise, we take vitamins, and we get our blood tested repeatedly to see how we are doing. However, in our enthusiasm to achieve the highest level of good health, we often have a tendency to overdo it, and particularly to overlook the positive nutritional value of foods available to us, concentrating instead on the negative aspects.

Understanding the whole subject of cholesterol intake, particularly where cholesterol comes from and how it affects our health and well-being, as well as the nutritional values of red meat, will give you a sensible approach to designing your daily food intake.

Recently I calculated the cholesterol I had consumed during my evening meal:

The soup had 55 milligrams of cholesterol,
The bread 12 milligrams, the butter 60 milligrams,
The salad none, but the dressing had 65 milligrams,
The 4-ounce filet had 75 milligrams,
The asparagus had none, but the butter had 50 milligrams,
The potato with sour cream, butter, and fixings had 90 milligrams,
Dessert added another 45 milligrams.

The total came to 452 milligrams of cholesterol, 152 milligrams more than the recommended daily allowance. Even if this cholesterol breakdown means nothing to you, you can readily see that in the context of a full meal, the cholesterol was really hidden in the garnishes on the so-called good foods, not in the red meat as we are too often led to believe.

Another interesting point to consider is that while the beef filet represented only 16 percent of my total cholesterol intake, it provided 60 percent of my recommended daily protein and 25 percent of my daily iron needs.

At long last we can all sit back and read this informative book and relax about putting beef back into our lives. Chriss McNaught has taken the "dubious" beef— long the victim of bad press where cholesterol is concerned— and has exposed some of the myths about beef and cholesterol. Believing in this American favorite, she has developed ways in which we can enjoy our beloved beef and still manage our cholesterol level, our weight, and our overall nutritional requirements.

With a moderate and sensible approach, this book shows that beef can be an integral part of anyone's diet.

The key to good nutrition and overall good health is *moderation.* The National Research Council has recently published its latest dietary recommendations which stressed the advantage of moderation in diet and exercise. Paramount among the recommendations, however, was that fat (and consequently cholesterol) intake be reduced to 30 percent of the total daily caloric intake. But it is important to note that the recommendation says "reduce" not "eliminate." Thus, in following the advice of the NRC, moderation is the guideline.

Diet books come and go. Many people have benefitted from one or the other approach, while others continue their struggle to lose weight, control their blood sugar and/ or cholesterol levels, and acquire and maintain physical fitness. What most people do not understand is that to change their state of health, they must also change their lifestyle and life-long eating patterns.

Thanks to medical discoveries, improved living conditions, and healthful practices, our life expectancy continues to lengthen. Can we increase our life expectancy even more by making further lifestyle and dietary changes? Current medical evidence actually suggests that this is not likely, but at the very least, proper management of diet and lifestyle will, in particular, decrease the occurrence of heart problems. And it is with the heart problems that cholesterol enters the debate.

Because we are blessed with an active scientific community, our understanding of cholesterol has greatly increased. The section in this book on Facts about Cholesterol gives a thorough, but easily understood explanation about cholesterol. The important points to remember about cholesterol are the following:

1. Cholesterol comes from eating fat from animal sources (including the fat in dairy products, meat, and eggs). It is also manufactured in the body and flows in the blood stream.

2. If the amount of cholesterol flowing through the blood stream is too great, excess amounts adhere to the lining of the arteries. These deposits cause a gradual narrowing of the arteries, which can lead eventually to atherosclerosis, the cause of angina, heart attacks, and even sudden death.

3. The deposit of cholesterol on the inside of the arteries takes a long time to reach dangerous levels.

Because the accumulation of the cholesterol deposits is a long process, it stands to reason that developing a proper diet and exercise program early would be most effective, but as with any health-related program, it is never too late to begin. (It should be noted also that nutrition is not the only factor affecting heart problems. Other factors include smoking, high blood pressure, diabetes, and gender.)

The build-up of cholesterol deposits is a slow process, and with dietary changes we may not feel any immediate change for the better. However, there is much scientific evidence to indicate that the incidence of heart disease can be lowered by these changes and reduced cholesterol levels, as well as routine exercise programs. Furthermore, as the kind and amount of fat intake in the diet is altered, cholesterol present in the bloodstream may begin to pick up cholesterol deposits on the walls of the arteries, thereby reversing the trend towards atherosclerosis.

If cholesterol is a part of our diet, and it obviously has been since man began to eat meat, can it be all bad? If we completely eliminate cholesterol from our diet we can potentially harm our bodies. We know that cholesterol plays an important part as building blocks in the manufacturing of certain hormones, vitamins, and cell wall structures. Thus, despite its bad reputation, cholesterol is still an essential part of our dietary needs. Although the body does produce its own cholesterol, it does not do so in sufficient amounts to satisfy the total body requirements.

The current consensus indicates that at cholesterol levels of greater than 200 milligrams, the relative risk of coronary artery disease begins to increase and does so more significantly at levels of greater than 240 milligrams.

The nutritional program in this book underlines the principle of good sense and moderation in a well-balanced program. This book does not promise overnight success, but it does provide a program than anyone can "live with" year after year. Good health and good nutrition do not mean that you cannot enjoy excellent and varied meals. Chriss McNaught's recipes suit every need from family meals, to individual luncheons, to large parties. The cholesterol is not missed in any of these tasty dishes. And they are all prepared with beef!

As a warning before beginning any dietary program, and especially if major cholesterol or health problems exist such as diabetes or renal failure, consult your physician prior to starting this or any other dietary modification. It is also important to have a baseline lipid profile (cholesterol test) taken so that you can monitor the fluctuations, and positive changes, in your cholesterol level.

Approach your dietary changes with enthusiasm but also with intelligent moderation. Establish goals that are appropriate for you. Develop a positive attitude towards your own good health and enjoy!

Enrique Alfaro, M.D.
Board Certified Internist
Member
American Medical Association
Cholesterol Education Staff

September, 1989

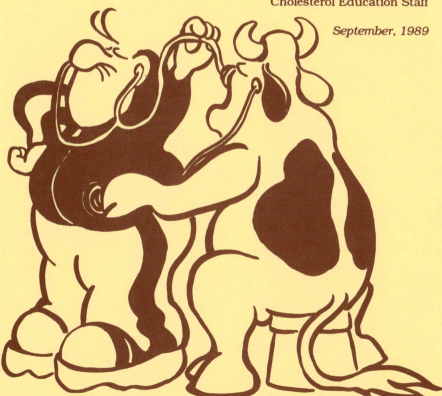

Introduction

Recently a friend of mine asked me what my qualifications were for writing a "Dietary Management Cook Book." Inasmuch as saying "an overweight husband" seemed a little unkind, I really was baffled. However, on thinking it over, I realized that like millions of women, I was eminently qualified, a conclusion I reached based entirely on the number of meals I have prepared. Actually, I feel I have produced twice as many meals as some women. When our children were younger, I made two separate dinners each evening. It was impossible to judge when my husband Ross would be finished with his day (he is an orthopedic surgeon), so I made one meal for the children and another one for Ross. That is when I discovered how versatile beef is, and how quickly beef can be turned into delicious, nutritious entrees.

Until a few years ago, we lived in large cities and were dependent upon food basics that were available in supermarkets. Over the years I came to rely on the consistent quality of beef. This is how beef became the central focus of our menus. When we moved to a more rural area, we had hopes of raising our own beef. But our one and only experiment with "Mr. Sam," the steer who turned out to be a bull, and not a friendly one at that, quickly changed our minds. We decided to leave beef production to the professionals.

However, if Ross had not seen a picture of himself sitting on a train, I would never have started changing my method of cooking or compiling the recipes in this book. But, the picture did it. Ross did look remarkably like a "pear" wearing plaid shorts. About the same time, I became aware of cholesterol and the health problems associated

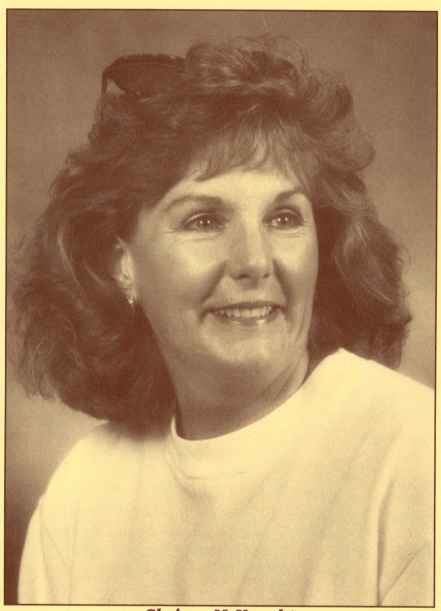

Chriss McNaught

with it. I was certain (and the baseline tests confirmed my suspicions) that Ross had an elevated blood cholesterol level. I was convinced that this was due at least in part to my cooking style, which relied heavily on butter, eggs, rich sauces, and other things generally associated with cholesterol-related problems.

My first trip to the bookstore to research cholesterol confirmed my worst suspicions: everything we enjoyed eating was wrong. Worse still was Ross's refusal to adapt to a diet without beef as its main component. Eventually I did find a grand total of 17 cholesterol-reduced beef recipes, but they did not begin to fit my criteria for exciting eating.

The only alternative that seemed to present itself was to develop my own recipes, and the only problem with this plan was that I had no experience in reducing calories or in reducing cholesterol, my expertise was in the opposite direction.

Initially, I took all our family favorites and altered them to reduce calories, cholesterol, and saturated fats. The amazing part was that my family did not object, in fact they did not even notice. However, as Ross began (for the first time in his life) to lose weight, and as he continued to change shape, everyone became increasingly interested in my efforts. Ross has now lost 30 pounds.(I have only lost 15.) We have both been able to maintain our reduced weight without being hungry or without feeling deprived. The proof has also appeared on Ross's cholesterol level. Through dietary management, it has dropped 35 points.

All in all, it has been a remarkably simple process. We are both proud of our success and our new shapes. While I still intend to lose 10 more pounds, Ross has reached his ideal weight, and it has all happened in under six months.

When friends asked me to write an outline of our program for them, it did not seem like a major project. However, as I became increasingly aware of the misconceptions relative to cholesterol and beef, I felt I had a responsibility to overweight beef lovers everywhere to share the simple formula of our success.

I am *not* an expert on the subject of dietary management or cholesterol, and if the introduction by Dr. Alfaro and the overview I have included create questions for you,

I would suggest visiting with your doctor. There are also many excellent detailed books available on the subject of cholesterol.

My goal was to develop exciting and tasty recipes that make eating fun while they also follow the guidelines established by the American Heart Association for good nutrition and a healthy heart. We love these recipes, and know you will, too. After you have tried them, I would like to hear from you; suggestions are always welcome. Also, please share your success with me as I would love to know that the plan worked for others also.

What follows is the philosophy that we found successful in reducing our weight and lowering our blood cholesterol level. I most certainly hope it works for you, too. Remember, beef really does build beautiful bodies.

Chriss McNaught
Cedar City, Utah
September, 1989

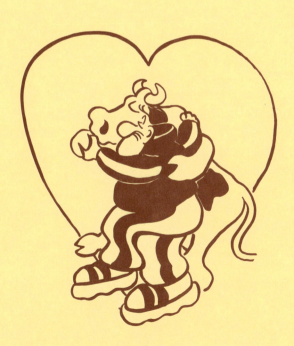

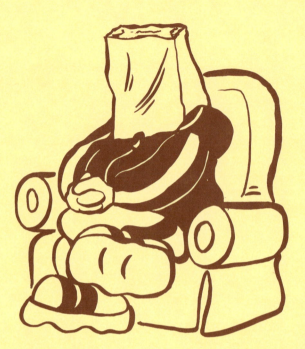

"You are what you eat," or worse, if you're a cartoonist, you are what you draw! And that's what happened to Jerry Palen, nationally syndicated cartoonist of the popular cartoon series STAMPEDE." I made it to age 40 and decided ENOUGH! I'd dieted, pushed up, sat up for the last time. If a guy can make it to 40 he ought to be able to relax, stop exercising, and eat what he wants."

"What happened in the next few years wasn't a pretty sight. I started looking like a cross between my own cartoon character ELMO and Sgt. Snorkle of Beetle Bailey."

"One day I was convinced I was having a heart attack. The tests from the hospital were grim." The doctor's diagnosis – "You've got high blood pressure, you're out of shape, and you're FAT!" The doctor's prescription – "You've got to lose weight, you've got to exercise!"

"I became the character in BEEF LOVER'S GUIDE. I didn't like chicken, nor fish, but I do like beef. So I started exercising and watching what I ate. Today I've lost my extra pounds, my blood pressure is down, my cholesterol is good, and I'm eating right. If Robert Redford was bald he'd look just like me!"

Jerry Palen

A Note about the Dietary Analyses of the Recipes

Dietary analysis was carried out by
Trisha Dobson, R.D.
Bachelor of Science with emphasis in Medical Dietetics.
Utah State University, Logan, Utah.
Member of the American Dietetic Association
Currently working as chief dietician,
Valley View Medical Center
Cedar City, Utah

All recipes in this book were analyzed by
The Nutritionist III Program
developed by
N^2 Computing
3040 Commercial Street SE, Suite 240
Salem, Oregon 97302

Nutritionist III is an Interactive Graphics Diet Analysis Program designed for professional and educational use. This computer program calculates nutritive analyses of single foods or combinations of foods that may be classified as recipes, meals, menus, or complete diets. Analyses include Weight and Percent of Recommended Dietary Allowances (RDA) for 58 nutrients including trace elements and amino acids. In addition, the proportion of protein, carbohydrate, fat, and alcohol contained in a food, meal, or diet as a percentage of the total caloric value is indicated.

For the purposes of this Book, analyses of the caloric, fat, saturated fat, and cholesterol content of each recipe was analyzed by this computer program, and those amounts are printed with each recipe.

This program is widely used in hospitals throughout the United States and came to the author's attention by its use in the LDS Hospital in Salt Lake City, Utah, and the Valley View Medical Center in Cedar City, Utah.

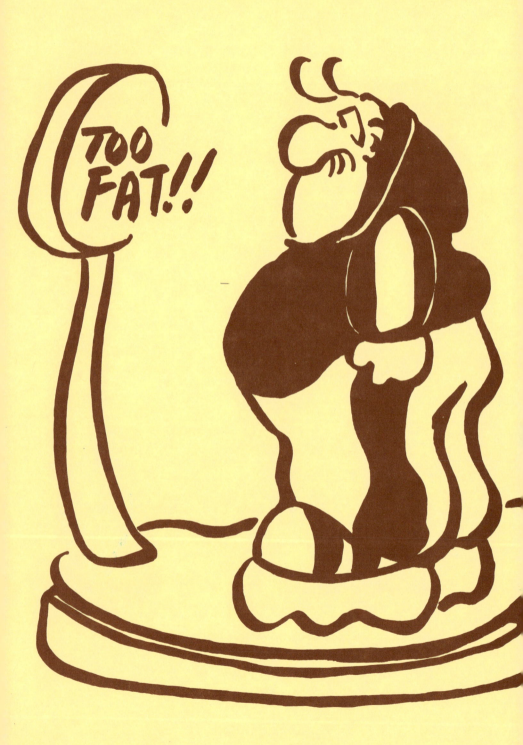

Begin a New Lifestyle

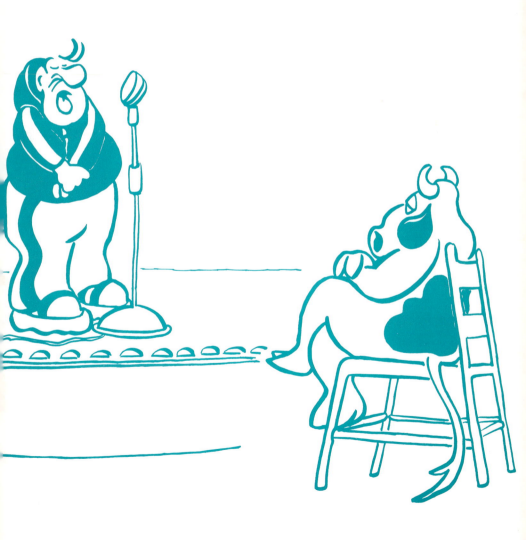

Develop a Philosophy

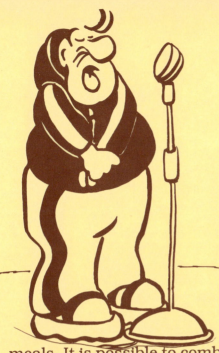

I believe that the secret to success in any situation is your own attitude. The secret to a successful diet is *mind* power, not *will* power.

Choosing foods for a balanced, healthy diet does not mean eliminating the pleasure of good food and exciting meals. It is possible to combine a wide variety of delicious foods in a way that is dietarily sound and lower in calories and cholesterol. Inasmuch as high blood pressure, obesity, clogged arteries, heart disease, and elevated blood cholesterol levels are all diet-related problems, it is important to develop eating patterns that reduce risk and promote good health.

Successful dieting should be a gradual process and done with the intention of making a permanent change in eating patterns. Changing a lifetime of eating habits takes determination but, above all, requires a *positive attitude*.

Calorie counting is just one aspect of controlling our weight. Sodium awareness is another. Reducing the amount of fat in our diet also produces a series of benefits.

Virtually every industry and association in the United States has issued guidelines for healthy eating. However, the American Heart Association guidelines for Healthy American Adults are the most widely accepted ones to follow for the prevention of cardiovascular diseases. But following these, or any dietary guidelines, is easier said than done.

While anyone can tell you what you should eat and should not eat, I believe the most important thing is to establish a personal philosophy that makes you want to achieve your goals.

Remain in Contol
My Personal Program for Dietary Success

♥ **Eliminate the word "diet" from your vocabulary.**
Replace it with "weight management."

♥ **Manage your weight effectively.**
You want to be in control. Accept the responsibility for your own health and weight. Do it for yourself.

♥ **Take credit for your own success.**
Be proud of the new you. Share your success with family and friends. It will have a positive effect on your own self-esteem.

♥ **Develop a system of personal positive reinforcement.**
Pep talks to yourself, notes on the refrigerator announcing how many pounds are gone. Use whatever motivates you and keeps your spirits up.

♥ **Monitor your eating habits.**
Be critical, but stress positive changes.

♥ **Short-term goals, stepping stones to an ultimate goal.**
Make sure your goals are reasonable (2 pounds a week weight loss is an appropriate goal for most people).

♥ **Establish a reward system for each goal.**
Because weight loss may vary, establish time frame goals.

♥ **Develop an exercise program which you enjoy**.
If your exercise program is burdensome, you will soon abandon it. Plan to exercise at a time that is reasonable and fits well with your daily schedule, thus helping to make it easy to maintain.

♥ **Do not weigh every day.**
There is a three-day delay before what you eat affects your weight, and daily weight checks often prove more disappointing and frustrating than encouraging.

♥ **Remain in control.**
That is the most important rule. Remember, it is your body and your own good health.

The
American Heart Association
Guidelines for Healthy Eating

1. Total fat intake should be less than 30% of calories.

2. Saturated fat intake should be less than 10% of calories.

3. Polyunsaturated fat intake should not exceed 10% of calories.

4. Cholesterol intake should not exceed 300 milligrams per day.

5. Carbohydrate intake should constitute 50% or more of calories, with emphasis on complex carbohydrates.

6. Protein intake should provide the remainder of the calories [less than 20% of total calorie intake].

7. Sodium intake should not exceed 3000 milligrams per day.

8. Alcoholic consumption should not exceed 1-2 ounces of ethanol per day. Two ounces of 100 proof whiskey, 8 ounces of wine, or 24 ounces of beer each contain 1 ounce of ethanol.

9. Total calories should be sufficient to maintain the individual's recommended body weight.

10. A wide variety of foods should be consumed.

Guidelines taken from "Dietary Guidelines for Healthy American Adults,"
©American Heart Association, 1988.

Weight Management

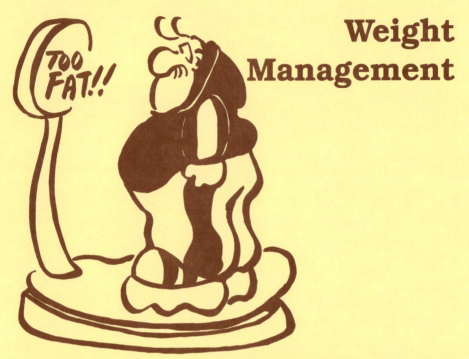

Today there is an ever-increasing focus on weight management. It is one part of the new awareness of the relationship between good health, proper diet, and adequate exercise. It is important to determine your own optimum weight and to develop a plan to achieve your weight goal.

♥ **Understand how weight is reduced**

♥ **Analyze your own eating patterns**

♥ **Keep records to monitor your patterns and to track your progress**

♥ **Develop your own weight management program
(formerly called a diet)**

The Ideal
Weight Management Program

♥ **Flexible**
Weight management is *not* an all or nothing situation.

♥ **In tune with our contemporary life style**

♥ **Realistic**

♥ **Based on an understanding of healthy eating and sound nutritional values**
It is the foundation for a healthy, vigorous life.

♥ **A permanent plan**
It has been proven repeatedly that the most satisfactory weight reduction plan is a calorie reduction plan resulting in slow, gradual weight loss which leads eventually to a full maintenance program.

♥ **A nutrient-dense vs. calorie-dense food plan**
A baked potato is nutrient dense, but French fries are calorie dense.

♥ **Full of variety**
50 nutrients are needed by our bodies on a daily basis for growth, maintenance, and repair. No one food group contains all the necessary nutrients in the required amounts. Therefore a wide variety of foods from different food categories should be consumed daily. All foods contain calories, but we should strive for nutrient dense food combinations.

The Basic Philosophy of Weight Loss

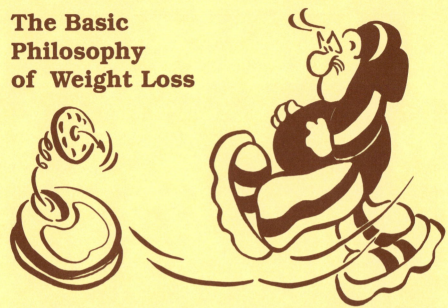

Until recently, I did not realize that it was possible to sum up the facts relative to weight loss and weight control in one paragraph; but the facts are simple, although not quite so simple to put into practice.

A pound of body fat contains about 3500 calories. To lose one pound of fat, you must burn 3500 calories more than you consume. The reverse is also true: if you eat 3500 calories more than you burn, you will gain one pound of body weight.

If you burn 500 calories a day more than you eat, you will lose one pound in 7 days. Thus, if you normally burn 2000 calories a day and maintain a 1500 calorie a day diet, you will lose 1 pound per week. Alternately, you may continue to eat 2000 calories per day and increase your exercise to maximize your calorie burn at 2500 calories a day and thereby achieve the same results.

No matter which way you approach weight loss, the best results seem to be achieved when you establish your target weight, eat less calories than is required to maintain that weight, and increase your exercise level.

Note: When you begin a weight-reduction diet, you may lose weight more rapidly at first, primarily due to existing water retention.

Target Your Weight
Steps to getting started

♥ **Determine your frame size**
A simple method is to take the middle finger and thumb of your left hand and place them around your right wrist. If they do not meet, your frame is large. If they just touch, your frame is medium, and if they over-lap your frame is small.

♥ **Determine your activity level**

♥ **Target your ideal weight**

♥ **Select your ideal calorie intake level**

♥ **Develop a management plan that suits you**

♥ **BEGIN**

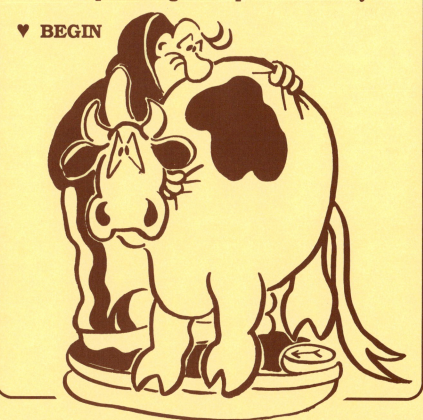

10   Begin a New Lifestyle

Table 12
Desirable Weights for Men and Women

Height (with Shoes)	Weight (In Indoor Clothing) Small Frame	Medium Frame	Large Frame
Men			
5 ft. 2 in.	128-134 lbs.	131-141 lbs.	138-150 lbs.
5 ft. 3 in.	130-136 lbs.	133-143 lbs.	140-153 lbs
5 ft. 4 in.	132-138 lbs.	135-145 lbs.	142-156 lbs.
5 ft. 5 in.	134-140 lbs.	137-148 lbs.	144-160 lbs.
5 ft. 6 in.	136-142 lbs.	139-151 lbs.	146-164 lbs.
5 ft. 7 in.	138-145 lbs.	142-154 lbs.	149-168 lbs.
5 ft. 8 in.	140-148 lbs.	145-157 lbs.	152-172 lbs.
5 ft. 9 in.	142-151 lbs.	148-160 lbs.	155-176 lbs.
5 ft. 10 in.	144-154 lbs.	151-163 lbs.	158-180 lbs.
5 ft. 11 in.	146-157 lbs.	154-166 lbs.	161-184 lbs.
6 ft. 0 in.	149-160 lbs.	157-170 lbs.	164-188 lbs.
6 ft. 1 in.	152-164 lbs.	160-174 lbs.	168-192 lbs.
6 ft. 2 in.	155-168 lbs.	164-178 lbs.	172-197 lbs.
6 ft. 3 in.	158-172 lbs.	167-182 lbs.	176-202 lbs.
6 ft. 4 in.	162-176 lbs.	171-187 lbs.	181-207 lbs.
Women			
4 ft. 10 in.	102-111 lbs.	109-121 lbs.	118-131 lbs.
4 ft. 11 in.	103-113 lbs.	111-123 lbs.	120-134 lbs.
5 ft. 0 in.	104-115 lbs.	113-126 lbs.	122-137 lbs.
5 ft. 1 in.	106-118 lbs.	115-129 lbs.	125-140 lbs.
5 ft. 2 in.	108-121 lbs.	118-132 lbs.	128-134 lbs.
5 ft. 3 in.	111-124 lbs.	121-135 lbs.	131-147 lbs.
5 ft. 4 in.	114-127 lbs.	124-138 lbs.	134-151 lbs.
5 ft. 5 in.	117-130 lbs.	127-141 lbs.	137-155 lbs.
5 ft. 6 in.	120-133 lbs.	130-144 lbs.	140-159 lbs.
5 ft. 7 in.	123-136 lbs.	133-147 lbs.	143-163 lbs.
5 ft. 8 in.	126-139 lbs.	136-150 lbs.	146-167 lbs.
5 ft. 9 in.	129-142 lbs.	139-153 lbs.	149-170 lbs.
5 ft. 10 in.	132-145 lbs.	142-156 lbs.	152-173 lbs.
5 ft. 11 in.	135-148 lbs.	145-159 lbs.	155-176 lbs.
6 ft. 0 in.	138-151 lbs.	148-162 lbs.	158-179 lbs.

Source: Prepared by the Metropolitan Life Insurance Company, 1983.

25 Tips to
Successful Weight Control

1. **Follow the American Heart Association nutritional guidelines.**

2. **Do not try to change all your behaviors at once.** You will have a much better chance of success if the changes are gradual.

3. **Chart your diet progress.**

4. **Read labels.** Information on labels keeps you in control of what you are eating.

5. **Plan your meals as a daily unit**, making sure all nutritional requirements are met.

6. **Don't skip meals**, especially breakfast.

7. **Eat slowly**, 20 to 30 minutes per meal.

8. **Reduce portion size.**

9. **Eat a variety of foods.**

10. **Eat everything in moderation.**

11. **Do not feel compelled to finish your portion** if you already feel satisfied, and *do not* have second helpings.

12. **Use liquid to control your hunger**, thus allowing you to make better food choices. 8 glasses of water per day is recommended.

13. **Begin your meal with a carbohydrate.** This lessens fat cravings.

12   Begin a New Lifestyle

14. **Eat breakfast at home.** It tends to be more calorie-wise and has a lower percentage of fat.

15. **Attempt to make lunch your largest meal** with a lighter meal for supper.

16. **Do a thorough kitchen cupboard cleaning,** eliminating all calorie-dense foods.

17. **Prepare meals using basic ingredients.** It helps you avoid hidden sodium and calories.

18. **Substitute low-fat, low-calorie ingredients**.

19. **Convert your favorite recipes into a low-fat, low-calorie version.**

20. **Select the appropriate cooking method** with an eye to reducing fat.

21. **Use artistic presentation.** Vary colors, textures, and temperatures as this satisfies other senses.

22. **Add seasonings** Use herbs, spices, vinegar, lemon juice, and garlic (but not salt!) to make meals more exciting.

23. **If you use alcohol, be moderate.**

24. **Strive for an energy balance.** Calories taken in should equal bodily function and physical activity needs on a maintenance diet.

25. **Enjoy an exercise program.**

26. **Develop a hobby.** It will distract you during difficult periods.

Exercise

To Be of Optimum Benefit Your Exercise Program Must Suit your Lifestyle. It Must be Convenient and It Absolutely Must be Fun!

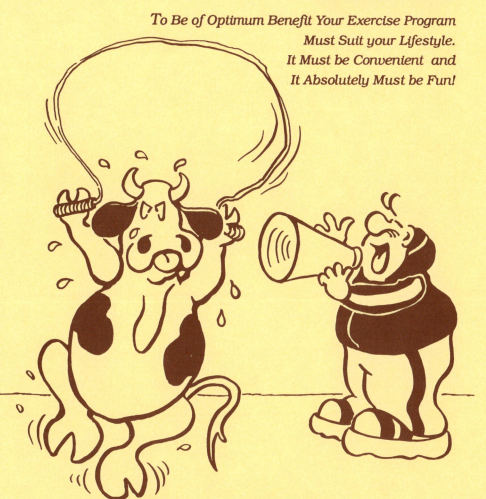

The benefits of exercise are immense

♥ Exercise controls weight by burning excess calories.

♥ Exercise speeds up the body's metabolism and increases the body's ability to burn fat for fuel, not only during the activity period but afterwards as well.

♥ Exercise has a calming effect which often curbs the appetite resulting in the consumption of fewer calories.

14   Begin a New Lifestyle

♥ Exercise increases "good" cholesterol and decreases "bad" cholesterol and helps control elevated blood pressure (hypertension) and related stress levels by controlling weight and by burning excess calories.

♥ Exercise is doing something nice for yourself, it creates a feeling of well being, produces relaxation benefits, helps occupy your free time, and it improves your self-image because you are in charge of doing something positive for your own good health.

Remember, your exercise program should be suited to your own needs. Be sure to begin slowly, and proceed with moderation. If you are over 40 or have any health related problems be sure to consult your physician.

Exercise Reduces Risk of Heart Disease

Exercise makes the heart stronger by making the heart muscle work more efficiently.

Here's how it works!

♥ Regular exercise causes electrical and chemical signals to stimulate the heart, as a result the heart pumps more quickly and forcefully. As the heart grows stronger, it pumps more blood, both more effectively and more efficiently.

♥ Muscles throughout the body become more efficient at extracting oxygen from the blood, further reducing the demand on the heart.

♥ Collateral circulation is increased and therefore more blood is delivered to and from the heart, increasing the hearts supply of oxygen and other essential nutrients.

A conditioned heart muscle functions less strenuously and more effectively.

Mean Heights and Weights and Recommended Energy Intake

	Age	Pounds	Energy needs*
Males	11-14	99	2700 (2000-3700)
	15-18	145	2800 (2100-3900)
	19-22	154	2900 (2500-3300)
	23-50	154	2700 (2300-3100)
	51-75	154	2400 (2000-2800)
	76+	154	2050 (1650-2450)
Females	11-14	101	2200 (1500-3000)
	5-18	120	2100 (1200-3000)
	9-22	120	2100 (1700-2500)
	23-50	120	2000 (1600-2400)
	51-75	120	1800 (1400-2200)
	76+	120	1600 (1200-2000)

*The energy expenditures are for persons whose activity levels are sedentary. (The values in parentheses are relative to the increased or decreased activity levels.)

The data in this table has been assembled from the observed median heights and weights of adults.

From: Recommended Dietary Allowances, Revised 1980. Food and Nutrition Board, National Academy of Sciences-National Research Council, Washington, D.C.

How to Find Your Ideal Weight
The Freeman Formula

This simple formula developed by Dr. Richard Freeman, Vice-Chairman of Medicine, at the University of Wisconsin in Madison is an easy way to determine your ideal weight.

The ideal female weight is 100 pounds for the first 5 feet of height, plus 5 pounds for each additional inch.

The formula for a male is 106 pounds for the first 5 feet of height, plus 6 pounds for each additional inch.

Frame size impact is calculated by adding 10% of the ideal base weight to the total, while a person of small frame may subtract 10%.

Activity Levels
(see chart on previous page)

Very Sedentary
Limited activity. Most time spent sitting, reading, or watching television. Some slow walking.

Sedentary
Includes fishing, skeet shooting, target shooting, motor boating, horseback riding, driving a car, walking, and limited slow jogging.

Moderately Active
Includes golf, sailing, skating, aerobic dancing, bowling, pleasure skiing, lawn mowing, and badminton.

Active
Includes swimming, tennis, cross-country skiing, jogging (three times a week), ping pong, and wood chopping.

Very Active
Vigorous activities include running, competitive athletics, such as football, soccer, basketball, squash, and racquetball.

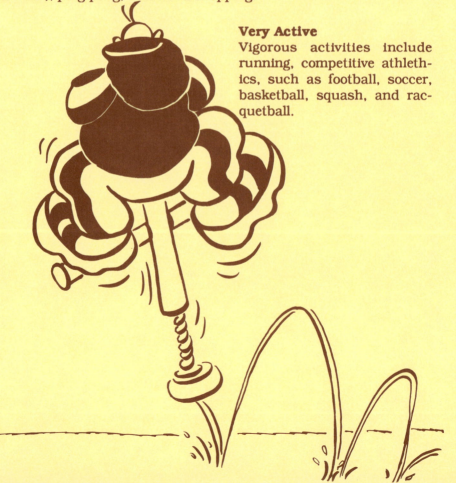

Calorie Expenditure of a Person Weighing 150 Pounds
Calculated Per Hour

Light Activity

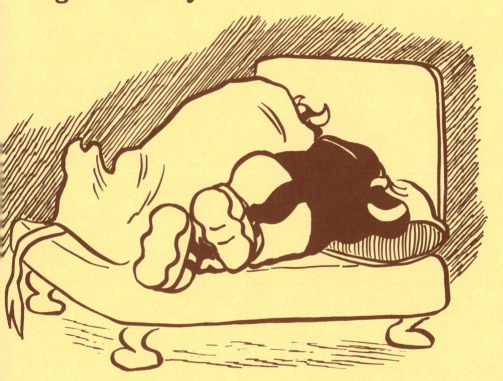

Lying down or sleeping	80
Sitting	100
Driving a car	120
Standing	140
Domestic work	180

Source: *USDA/USDHHS Dietary Guidelines.* Based on material prepared by Robert E. Johnson, M.D., Ph.D. and colleagues, University of Illinois.

Moderate Activity

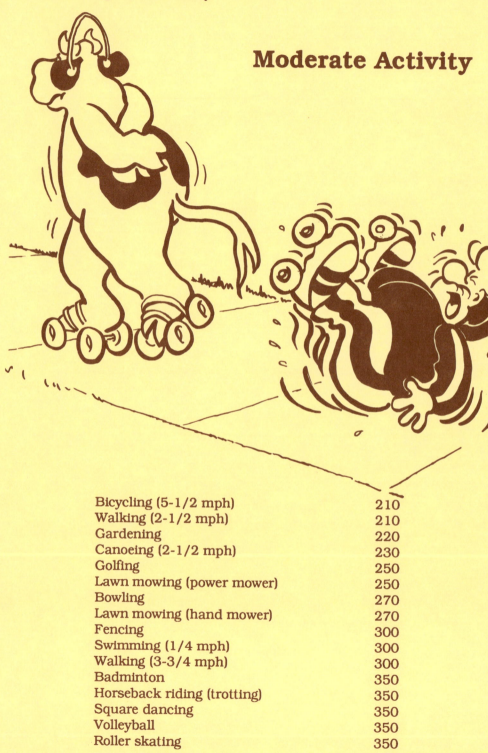

Bicycling (5-1/2 mph)	210
Walking (2-1/2 mph)	210
Gardening	220
Canoeing (2-1/2 mph)	230
Golfing	250
Lawn mowing (power mower)	250
Bowling	270
Lawn mowing (hand mower)	270
Fencing	300
Swimming (1/4 mph)	300
Walking (3-3/4 mph)	300
Badminton	350
Horseback riding (trotting)	350
Square dancing	350
Volleyball	350
Roller skating	350

Vigorous Activity

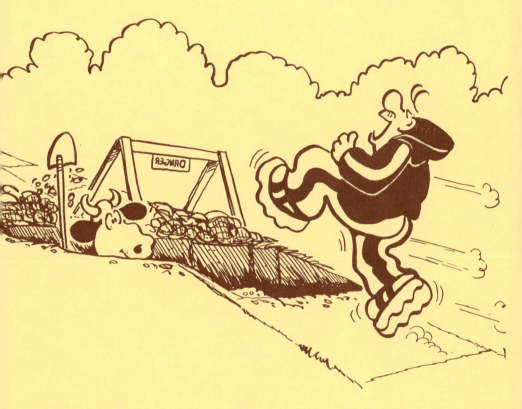

Table tennis	360
Ditch digging	400
Ice skating (10 mph)	400
Wood chopping	400
Tennis	420
Water skiing	480
Skiing (10 mph)	600
Squash and racquetball	600
Cycling (13 mph)	660
Running	900

20 Begin a New Lifestyle

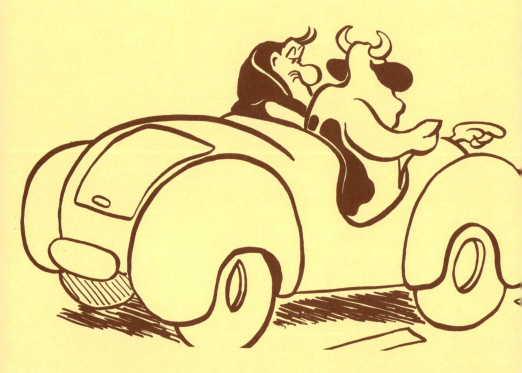

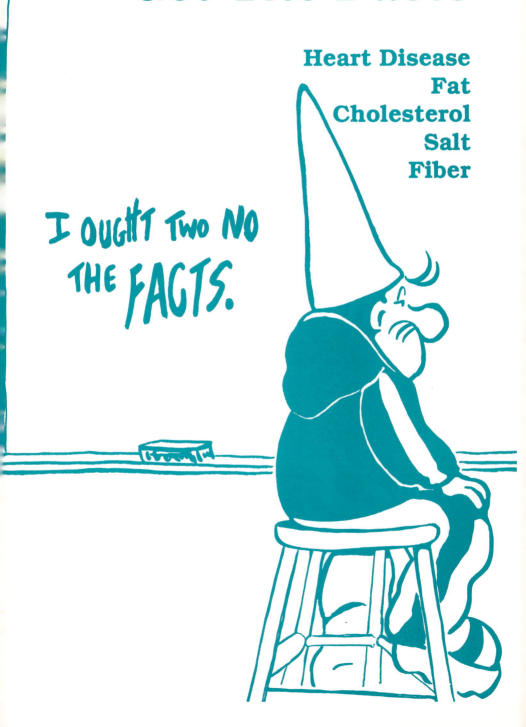

Facts About

Heart Disease

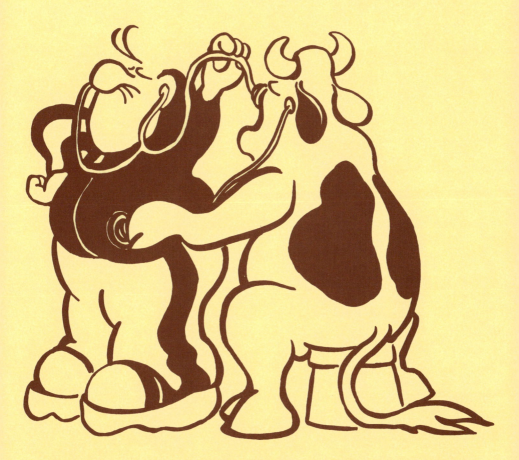

Atherosclerosis, arteriosclerosis, and the resulting heart-health problems are a leading cause of death in the United States. These conditions are commonly called *heart disease*. Heart disease is really a misnomer. The heart is not diseased; it is the blood supply to the heart which is impaired and causes heart-related problems, such as angina, stroke, and heart attack.

Know The Terms

♥ Plaque is the name given to the deposits of fibrous tissue, fat, cholesterol, and calcium which accumulates on the interior walls of the arteries.

♥ Atherosclerosis is the medical name for the build-up of plaque on artery walls. Atherosclerosis is a slow, progressive disease, sometimes not producing symptoms for 20 years or more. But the disease may suddenly materialize with serious, often fatal, complications, such as heart attack or stroke.

♥ Arteriosclerosis (commonly known as hardening of the arteries) is the condition in which plaques adheres to the inside walls of the arteries causing them to lose their elasticity, harden, and sometimes thicken, which in turn impairs the blood supply to the heart.

♥ Angina is the warning signal of a dangerous heart problem. When blood flow to the heart begins to be impaired, angina occurs. Angina is distinguished by spasmodic attacks of intense pain in the chest.

♥ Heart attack and stroke occur when the flow of blood to the heart is significantly impaired. A blood clot forms in the artery preventing the blood, oxygen, and nutrients from reaching the heart muscle.

Risk Factors Affecting Heart Disease

♥ Gender and genetics affect a person's potential-for heart disease.Women are less likey to develop atherosclerosis than men. Those with family histories of heart disease run a higher risk of developing the disease.

♥ Other risk factors which influence heart disease can be managed and controlled:

High blood cholesterol
Elevated blood pressure/hypertension
Smoking
Diabetes
Marked obesity
Lack of physical exercise

♥ The medical community generally agrees that a positive change in any of the risk factors affecting heart disease will begin to offset the severity of atherosclerosis. For example, modifying diet to consume less fat and fewer calories and exercising regularly are actions that can begin to reverse the build-up of plaque and lead directly to better health.

Facts About Fat

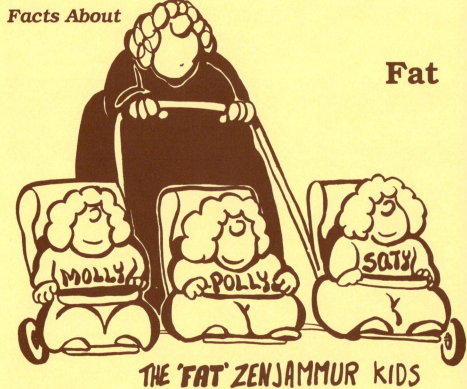

THE 'FAT' ZENJAMMUR KIDS

♥ Fat is an essential nutrient required by our bodies on a daily basis to maintain good health. It is one of the three basic food substances (the other two being protein and carbohydrate). Fat is needed to transport vitamins A, D, and E through the body.

♥ Fats add flavor to foods and create a sense of satisfaction (feeling of fullness).

♥ Fats are an excellent source of energy. They provide more calories per gram than carbohydrates.

♥ Fat is not only consumed through foods eaten, but is also produced in the body. When fat consumption exceeds the body's requirements, the body's fat cells store the excess. The result is extra body fat. Continued accumulation of fat will lead eventually to obesity.

Facts **27**

♥ Once formed, fat cells never die; they simply shrink and then wait for a state of caloric surplus to exist so that excess calories can be converted to fat.

♥ Fat that is consumed goes to the intestines where bile breaks it down into a form that the body can use. It then forms into a compound called lipoprotein (fat+protein) and is transported through the blood-stream to all body cells where the fat is either used to generate calories or is stored for later use.

♥ There is a direct relationship between the consumption of fat, specifically saturated fat, and the level of blood cholesterol.

♥ Reducing saturated fat consumption is the most effective dietary measure in reducing blood cholesterol levels. Eating less saturated fat reduces the chance of fatty deposits in the arteries; however, eating other fats will result in fatty deposits elsewhere.

♥ The American Heart Association recommends that daily fat intake should not exceed 30% of total caloric intake, and be divided equally between the three types of fat. Therefore, the allowance for saturated fat should never exceed 10% of the total caloric intake.

♥ The average person consumes more fat than is required. Cutting back on fat consumption is made more difficult because so many fat calories are hidden in the way foods are prepared. Understanding the different types of fat and where they are found is essential.

Understanding the Chemistry of Fat

Any discussion of the chemistry of fat is confusing unless you are a biochemist. But it is important to know enough chemistry to understand how fat works in the body.

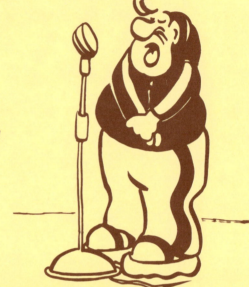

♥ Fat is the term commonly used for a group of chemical compounds called lipids. Lipids are made up of long chains of carbon atoms, like pearls on a string, to which hydrogen atoms are attached. These chains become fatty acid molecules, which often bind together with other molecules, in particular sugar (glycerol) to make glycerides, phosphates to make phospholipids, and nitrogen to make lecithin. These variations create the different kinds of fats.

♥ Fat does not dissolve in water. When it floats through the bloodstream, it sticks together and does not mix with the water. (Drop some cooking oil into a glass of water to see the effect.)

♥ Fat is generally classified into three groups: simple, compound, or associated fats. From the dietary point of view, the fats to study are simple fats, and those compounds which are associated, or carried along with the fat.

Know the Terms

♥ Simple Fat

Fat in food is made up mostly of neutral fat. The most common of these simple fats is triglycerides (a compound made up of three fatty acid molecules bound to glycerol).

♥ Compound Fat

These fats are more complex, containing phosphate and nitrogen, and are used up (rather than stored) by the body. They are needed in the make-up of cell structure, found in nerve tissue, and help transport fat through the body.

♥ Associated Fat

These "fats" are actually not fats at all, but are other compounds which dissolve in fat and thus become associated with fat. Such compounds are hormones, cholesterol, and vitamins.

♥ Saturated and Unsaturated Fats

The way in which the molecules in fatty acids bind to each other give the names of saturated, monounsaturated, and polyunsaturated fat. The more hydrogen molecules that are attached to carbons in the chain, the more saturated the fat. Saturated fat, therefore, has the maximum number of hydrogen molecules attached to each carbon molecule.

It is not necessary to understand the molecular structures. However, it is the structure of these compounds that influence how the fat breaks down, how it is transported, and what other compounds are found with it. It is important to know in which foods those fats are found and what research has told us about their role in good nutrition.

♥ **Saturated Fat.** Cholesterol is associated mainly with saturated fat. Saturated fats are found in all animal fat as well as in five vegetable fats: coconut oil, palm oil, palm kernel oil, cocoa butter, and hydrogenated vegetable oil. Saturated fats are generally solid at room temperature.

♥ **Monounsaturated Fat.** Current research indicates that monounsaturated fat lowers total blood cholesterol. In its make-up, it appears to have the ability to transport cholesterol out of the body. However, research is still inconclusive. Olive oil is the best source of monounsaturated fat.

♥ **Polyunsaturated Fat.** Cholesterol does not associate with this fat. Foods and vegetable oils which have no cholesterol may still contain fat in a polyunsatarated form. Polyunsaturated fats are liquid at room temperature.

Fat Trimming Tips

The American Heart Association recommends that fat intake not exceed 30% of total caloric consumption, and be divided equally between the three types of fat. The recommended allowance for saturated fat is 10% of daily calorie consumption.

Because so many foods contain fat, it is not possible to eliminate it from your diet by avoiding any one group of foods. However, by becoming aware of fat content and trimming it from many foods, it is possible to regulate fat consumption.

♥ Read labels carefully.

♥ Reduce amount of butter, margarine, and cooking oil.

♥ Choose lean cuts of meat.

♥ Trim all visible fat from meat portions.

♥ Always drain any liquid fat.

♥ Roast or grill meat on a rack, allowing fat to drain off during cooking.

♥ Use low-fat cooking methods, such as baking, steaming, poaching or boiling.

♥ De-fat meat drippings and broth before using.

♥ Rinse browned ground steak under hot water in a colander. Pat dry with paper towel.

Facts   31

♥ Use low-fat products whenever possible. For example, skim milk versus whole milk.

♥ Saute in wine, broth, water, or vinegar, using a non-stick pan.

♥ Eliminate rich sauces and gravies; substitute low-fat sauces or relishes.

♥ Keep salad dressings to a minimum.

♥ Use lemon juice and herbs on vegetables.

♥ Avoid convenience foods and commercially baked goods.

♥ Snack on fruits, vegetables, and unbuttered popcorn.

♥ Drink at least 8 glasses of water per day.

How to Figure the Percentage of Fat in Calories

It is essential to count fat (and particularly saturated fat) calories. Use the following formula to calculate what percentage fat your total calorie intake has been:

If 1 serving has 190 calories and 17 grams of fat

**Multiply the grams of fat by 9:
(17x9) = 153 calories.**

**Divide 153 by the total number of calories:
(153/190=80%).**

Thus, the calories in this serving contained 80% fat.

Percentage of Fat in Common Foods

Dairy Products

Cheddar cheese (2 oz.)	74%
Mozzarella cheese (2 oz.)	55%
Cheese spread (2 oz.)	65%
Cottage cheese (1/2 cup)	18%
Whole milk (1 cup)	48%
2% milk (1 cup)	34%
Skim milk (1 cup)	6%
Yogurt (2%, 1 cup)	25%
Ice cream (10%, 1 cup)	47%
Butter	99%
Heavy cream	96%
Sour cream	88%
Cream cheese	84%
Roquefort cheese	74%
American cheese	74%
Blue cheese	73%
Parmesan cheese	60%

Grains and Nuts

Whole wheat bread (1 slice)	15%
Rice, cooked (1/2 cup)	0%
oatmeal (1/2 cup)	12%
Granola (1/2 cup)	36%
Peanuts, dry roasted (1/2 cup)	78%
Peanut Butter (2 tbsp.)	76%

Vegetables and Fruits

Apple or pear	5%
Avocado	87%
Potato, baked	1%
French fries (20)	36%
Potato chips (20)	60%
Pinto beans, cooked (1/2 cup)	2%
Pork and beans (1/2 cup)	23%

Beef (3 oz.) 40%

Fish, Poultry, and Eggs

Roast beef, lean (4 oz.)	33%
Steak, untrimmed (4 oz.)	74%
Salami (4 oz.)	74%
Pork chop, lean (4 oz.)	53%
Turkey breast (4 oz.)	6%
Chicken, without skin (4 oz.)	19%
Chicken, with skin (4 oz.)	36%
Salmon (4 oz.)	35%
Shrimp (4 oz.)	7%
Liver (4 oz.)	42%
Egg	68%
Big Mac (McDonald's™)	53%

Fats and Dressings

Butter (1 tbsp.)	99%
Margarine (1 tbsp.)	99%
Vegetable oil (1 tbsp.)	100%
Mayonnaise (1 tbsp.)	100%
French dressing (2 tbsp.)	84%
Milk chocolate bar (1.2 oz.)	56%

Facts   33

Facts About

Cholesterol

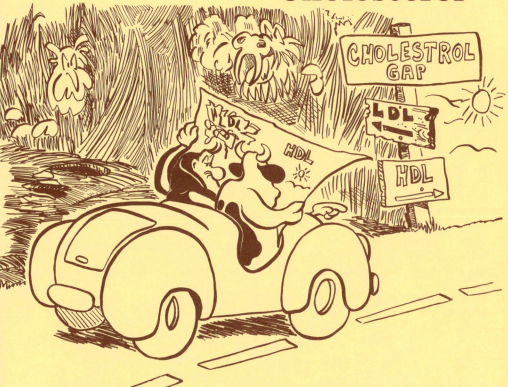

♥ Cholesterol is an organic chemical compound which is an essential part of all animal (including human) cell membranes. It is a necessary starting ingredient to make hormones, bile, and cell membranes in the body.

♥ Cholesterol is manufactured in the liver of animals (including humans) whether or not they eat saturated fats or cholesterol.

♥ Cholesterol is also taken into the body through consumption of fats from animal sources, including all meats and consumption of dairy products.

♥ Cholesterol is soluble in oils and fats, but not soluble in water. It is therefore found together with fats (associated fats), especially with saturated fats. When large amounts of saturated fats are consumed, blood cholesterol levels tend to rise.

♥ Cholesterol floats through the bloodstream attached to fat and protein in a compound called a lipoprotein.

♥ Elevated levels of cholesterol in the blood is a contributing factor in the development of atherosclerosis.

♥ Elevated high-risk cholesterol levels are usually caused by one of three reasons:
1. The body produces unusually large amounts of cholesterol,
2. The body does not eliminate excess cholesterol, or
3. Diet contains too much fat or cholesterol which the body is unable to utilize properly.

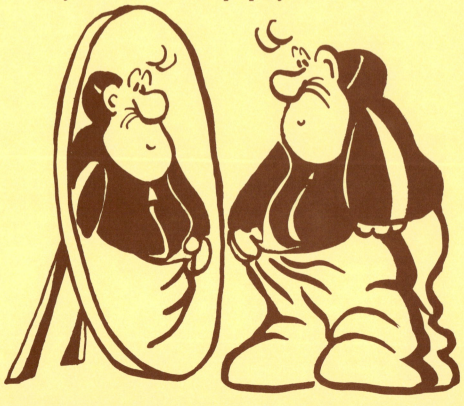

Facts   35

Know the Terms

♥ High Density Lipoprotein (HDL)
HDL is known as the "good cholesterol." It is not, however, cholesterol but is a durable, tightly bound lipoprotein which transports excessive cholesterol to the liver for processing and elimination from the body. In its rapid movement through the bloodstream, it will also absorb pieces of plaque build-up which are present on the linings of arteries and thus reverse the process of atherosclerosis. Therefore, the higher the HDL level, the greater the protection against atherosclerosis.

♥ Low Density Lipoprotein (LDL)
These lipoproteins are large, loosely bound, and not very stable. They are likely to break apart when excessive amounts of cholesterol are attached. When they break apart, they deposit cholesterol onto the artery walls, leading to the build-up of plaque in the arteries. High consumption of saturated fats leads to greater production of LDLs in the body. Research has shown that most people with high blood cholesterol levels have elevated LDL levels.

♥ Very Low Density Lipoprotein (VLDL)
This is the substance used by the liver to manufacture LDL; therefore, the higher the level of VLDL, the more LDL is produced by the liver.

♥ Triglycerides
These are simple fats, not lipoproteins. Because it is soluble in this type of fat, cholesterol is associated with triglycerides. Scientists have found that there is a relationship between elevated cholesterol levels and elevated triglyceride levels. Also, lowering the triglyceride level appears to lower the blood cholesterol level.

Note: The ratio between LDL and HDL is of extreme importance. The lower the ratio, the greater the risk, since there is then more LDL lining the arteries with plaque than there is HDL trying to keep the cholesterol away from the artery linings.

The Baseline Lipid Profile Test

A simple blood test can detemine whether a person's cholesterol level is too high. It is recommended that everyone take this test to establish a personal profile.

Knowing your own cholesterol level can help you make the necessary adjustments in diet and lifestyle to keep fat and cholesterol levels within acceptable ranges. Drug therapy is available for extreme cases.

The Baseline Lipid Profile Test will give you your levels of lipoproteins (HDL, LDL, and VLDL) and triglycerides. Together these components are used to determine your level of cholesterol.

Cholesterol Risk Levels

(according to the National Institutes of Health)

AGE	RECOMMENDED LEVEL	MODERATE RISK	HIGH RISK
2-19	Less than 170	170-185	Greater than 185
20-29	Less than 200	200-220	Greater than 220
30-39	Less than 220	220-240	Greater than 240
40+	Less than 240	240-260	Greater than 260

♥ **What the numbers mean**

Doctors give cholesterol levels in metric units, so that a cholesterol level of 200 actually means that there are 200 milligrams of cholesterol present in a sample of 1 deciliter of blood. One milligram is roughly the equivalent of 1/28,000th of an ounce and a deciliter is slightly more than 3 ounces.

Tips for Raising HDL Levels

Large amounts of High-Density Lipoproteins (HDL) in the bloodstream tend to lower cholesterol levels. Here are some tips to raise the HDL level and fight cholesterol:

* ♥ Eat a diet low in fats and cholesterol, and reduced in total calories.
* ♥ Reduce intake of saturated fat.
* ♥ Increase exercise.
* ♥ Maintain a healthy weight (overweight people are more likely to have higher levels of LDLs).
* ♥ Don't smoke. Nicotinic acid is known to stop the liver from manufacturing certain lipoproteins.

Cholesterol Trimming Tips

Daily recommended intake of cholesterol is 300 milligrams

♥ **Limit fat intake to 30% and all saturated fat to 10% of daily calorie intake.**
Limiting fat naturally reduces calorie and cholesterol intake.

♥ **Select lean meat portions and always trim all visible fat**.
Choose cooking methods which further reduce fat content, such as broiling, poaching, or grilling.

♥ **Add oat bran to your daily diet**.
This fiber whisks fats and cholesterol through the digestive system.

♥ **There is no cholesterol in plants.**
Fruits and vegetables make great snacks and complex carbohydrates are filling as well as nutritious.

♥ **Limit egg yolks to fewer than 3 per week**.
There is no limit on egg whites, as they contain no fat or cholesterol. Two egg whites may be substituted for 1 egg in many recipes.

38 Facts

"Establishing a low-fat, low-cholesterol diet can be easy if you follow a few simple guidelines."

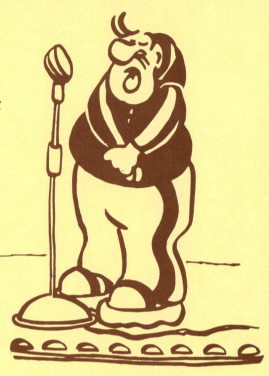

**4 or more servings
Vegetables and fruits, fruit juices, vegetable juices**

One serving is:
- 1/2 cup fruit or vegetable juice
- 1 med. (3") fruit or vegetable
- 1/2 cup cooked fruit or vegetable

**2 servings only
Fish, poultry, meat, dried beans and peas, nuts, and eggs**

One serving is:
- 2-3 ounces of meat, fish, or poultry

**4 or more servings
Breads, cereals, and starchy foods**

One serving is:
- 1 slice bread
- 1 cup dry cereal
- 1/2 cup cooked cereal
- 1/2 cup pasta, rice, noodles
- 2 graham crackers
- 1 cup popcorn (air popped)

**2 or more servings
Milk and cheese**

One serving is:
- one 8 ounce glass, low-fat or nonfat butter milk
- 1 ounce low-fat cheese
- one 1/3 cup low-fat Cottage cheese
- one 8 ounce carton low-fat yogurt

Facts About Salt

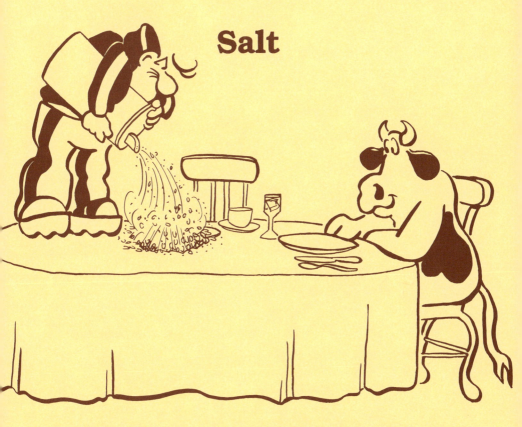

Understanding sodium is essential to positive weight management. There are two sources of sodium, hidden and unhidden. There are food items where you know (or can taste) that sodium is present, such as in the salt shaker, potato chips, soy sauce, salted nuts, salted popcorn, and bouillon cubes. It is certainly easy to be aware of and control eating these products.

Clearly it is not possible to eliminate salt from our diet, but knowing where it is hidden is the first step in monitoring it's use. The second step is changing your taste expectations and coming to enjoy the natural taste of food, and this can be done in conjunction with a growing appreciation for other seasonings, while limiting the use of salt.

Look for Hidden Salt

Bottled soft drinks
Fast foods
Commercial baked goods
Cake, cookie, and pancake mixes
Quick cooking instant cereals
Dry cereals
Canned vegetable or tomato juice
Canned tomato sauce, paste, and puree
Canned products, such as chili con carne
Catsup
Mustard
Pickles
Relish
Steak sauce
Some peanut butters
Fish packaged in oil
Processed meats (hotdogs, salami, etc.)
Ham
Bacon
Sausage
Dehydrated and frozen dinners
Dehydrated and frozen vegetables
Commercial salad dressings
Dehydrated soup and sauce mixes
Cheese and processed cheese spreads

Salt Trimming Tips

*The recommended daily allowance
of sodium is 3000 milligrams*

Don'ts

♥ Avoid using salt as a condiment at the table (removing the shaker altogether works well).

♥ Avoid obviously salty foods such as pickles and potato chips.

♥ Avoid fast foods.

♥ Avoid processed and frozen foods.

♥ Avoid commercially baked goods.

♥ Avoid commercial mixes.

♥ Avoid packaged snack food.

♥ Avoid sugar substitutes.

♥ Avoid bottled pop.

♥ Avoid quick cooking or instant cereals.

♥ Don't add salt when cooking.

♥ Do not add salt to meat, it delays browning and drains the moisture from the meat.

Do's

♥ Do think about the salt you are using. Remember, 1 teaspoon of salt equals 2300 milligrams, nearly a full day's allotment.

♥ Do read labels carefully.

♥ Do season foods with lemon juice, vinegar, herbs, spices, pepper, ginger, garlic (my favorite), onions, wine or Cajun spices.

♥ Do use low-sodium soy sauce, and Mrs. Dash™ seasonings are great.

♥ Do use lots of freshly ground pepper.

♥ Do use natural foods. Rather than sauces, use fresh fruit.

♥ Do make recipes from scratch because then you can control the amount of salt.

♥ Do decrease salt in recipes by one-half.

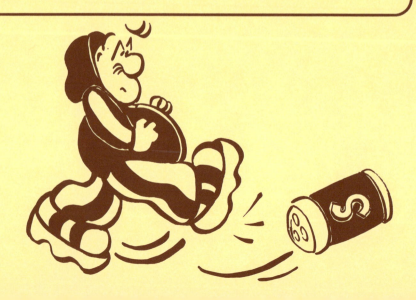

Facts About

Fiber

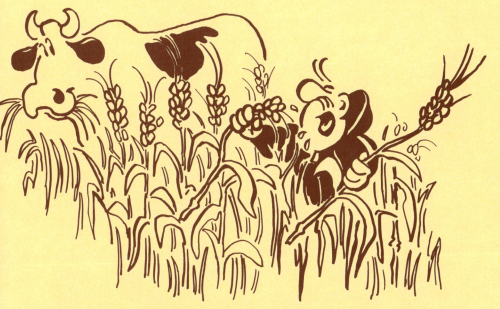

Fiber is a substance which is not digested or is only partially digested. Your grandmother called it "roughage". It is found in fruit, vegetables, cereals, and grains, and it is good for you. There are two types of fiber:

Insoluble Fiber
This fiber, found in whole grains and bran, does not dissolve in water, but rather absorbs water and swells. This swelling provides bulk and facilitates digestion. It is also widely accepted in the medical community that insoluble fiber may reduce the risk of colon-rectal cancer and diverticulitis by removing carcinogens and fat out of the intestine quickly. Some scientists believe high fiber foods decrease the possibility of absorption of calories and fat.

Soluble Fiber
This fiber, found in fruits, vegetables, and legumes, will dissolve in water, and helps to lower blood cholesterol and obesity by whisking fats and cholesterol through the digestive system. An added bonus is that soluble fiber creates a feeling of fullness. They are both nutritious and naturally low in calories and fat.

Put Fiber into Your Diet

♥ Eat 4 to 5 servings of fruit and vegetables per day.

♥ Eat edible skins of fruits and vegetables.

♥ Choose fruits or vegetables as snacks.

♥ Choose whole fruit over juices.

♥ Use whole wheat flour (substitute 1/2 whole wheat flour and 1/2 white flour in recipes).

♥ Choose whole wheat products when selecting bread products, pasta or crackers.

♥ Use whole wheat or unbleached flour when making waffles, pancakes; top with fresh fruit and low-fat yogurt instead of butter and syrup.

♥ Have bran muffins rather than prepared breakfast cereals.

♥ Choose breakfast cereals with at least 2 grams of fiber per serving.

♥ Add bran, whole wheat bread crumbs* or wheat germ to muffins, cereals, cookies, or meat loaf.

♥ Use regular oatmeal, not instant.

♥ Use brown rice instead of white rice.

♥ Add kidney beans to soups, salads, or casseroles.

♥ Add shredded carrots, zucchini, or other vegetables to soups, salads, casseroles, or spaghetti.

Note: Recent medical information confirms that oat bran (a soluble fiber) can help to reduce blood cholesterol levels, but it cannot offset the effects of a high cholesterol diet. It simply gives an extra boost to a low-fat, low-cholesterol diet.

*To make your own whole wheat bread crumbs, process 2 slices of whole wheat bread in a food processor or blender for 1 minute on high.

Adapting Your Own Recipes

Every family has favorite recipes and one of the best ways to ensure that your "new" weight management program works is to make it familiar and comfortable. Therefore it becomes necessary to find ways to change your favorite recipes, reducing the calories, sodium, and fat (particularly the saturated fat), while at the same time retaining the original flavor and texture. The diet department at your supermarket is a very good place to start; there are many products available that are readily interchangeable. Again, reading labels is important and learning to interpret the product claims is essential. But the most important skill to develop is to substitute low-fat, low-calorie, and low-sodium products for those with higher values.

Recipes can still be both tasty and exciting. The following is a brief list of easy substitutions to get you started.

When the Recipe calls for:	Use Instead:
Shortening or lard	Liquid vegetable oil
Butter	Margarine*
Butter for saute	Low-sodium broth or wine
Sour cream	Buttermilk
Whipping cream	Flavored low-fat yogurt
Whole milk	Skim milk
1 egg	2 egg whites
2 eggs	1 egg + 1 egg white

*Margarine and butter have the same fat content and caloric value, but margarine is made from vegetable oil and therefore has no cholesterol and reduced amounts of saturated fat.

46   Facts

Daily Menu Planning

1. Select food items and recipes you enjoy.
2. Enter the item or recipe and their values in the chart.
3. Add the values in each column and compare them to your daily allowance values.
4. Make any changes to fit the daily allowance.

Date:	Calories	Cholesterol	Saturated Fat	Fat
Breakfast				
Lunch				
Dinner				
Snacks				
Daily Total				
Daily Allowance				

Corraling Those
Beef Facts

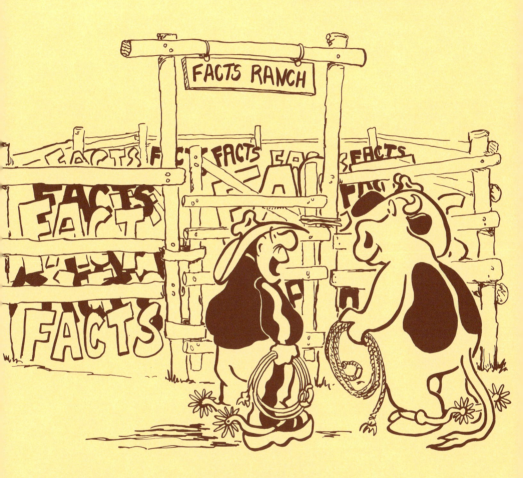

♥ FACT: Beef Is Low in Cholesterol
Three ounces of trimmed, cooked lean beef (from about 4 ounces raw beef) contain 76 milligrams of cholesterol. By comparison, the same amount of roasted chicken, with skin removed, also contains 76 milligrams. Pork contains 79 milligrams, flounder, 59 milligrams, shrimp, 129 milligrams, and turkey, 65 milligrams.

♥ FACT: Beef Falls Within AHA Guidelines
The American Heart Association recommends a limit of 300 milligrams of cholesterol per day. A 3-ounce serving of beef provides about 25% of this allowance.

FACT: Beef Is Part of a Low-Calorie Diet.
Three ounces of cooked, lean beef contains only 198 calories. Three ounces of roasted chicken, without skin, contains 162 calories; three ounces of fried chicken, with skin, contains 246 calories; and three ounces of pork contains 198 calories. Each 3-ounce serving of beef provides only 10 -12% of the calories in a 2000-calorie diet.

FACT: All Animal Fat is *NOT* Saturated Fat.
A cooked 3-ounce serving of trimmed beef contains 8.7 grams of total fat, of which less than half is saturated. A leaner cut, such as top round, contains 5.3 grams of total fat, of which about 2 grams are saturated.

FACT: Beef Contains The Nutrients for Good Health.
Ounce for ounce, beef is packed full of many good nutrients. For less than 200 calories per 3-ounce serving, beef's six leanest cuts supply the adult male with 27% of the daily recommended iron intake, 40% of the riboflavin (B-2), and 20% of the niacin, as well as 41% of the required protein.

FACT: Beef is the Best Food Source of Heme Iron.
Of special note is that sixty percent of the iron provided by beef is "heme iron," a type that is three to five times more easily absorbed by the body than non-heme iron, which is found in sources such as vegetables, cheese and eggs. Research studies with human subjects have shown that meat in a meal enhances the absorption of non-heme iron from other foods eaten at the same time.

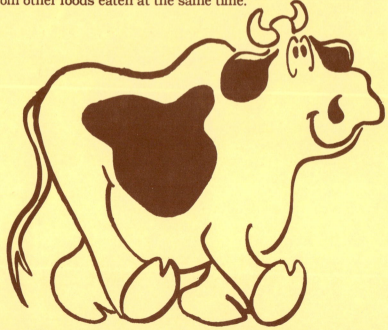

FACT: Beef is Safe.
According to USDA's 1986 figures, beef is one of the safest meats available. At the time of slaughter, beef contains no hazardous drug residues, nor any salmonellae contamination. Any contamination which may occur in beef comes with processing and handling.

FACT: Beef is Thoroughly Inspected.
Thousands of regulations guide each packing plant to ensure conditions of cleanliness. Beef packing and processing plants are operated under sanitation guidelines established by the U.S. Department of Agriculture (USDA) Food Safety and Inspection Service (FSIS). USDA or state meat inspectors are present during slaughter.

FACT: Beef Producers are Breeding Trimmer Animals.
Years of research and development have gone into the production of cattle with less body coverage of fat. That means that the fat one sees on the outside of the meat is not only being trimmed away, it is being bred away. It is also in this outside fat that saturated fat is most concentrated. The fat, or marbleing, that is present within the meat cut is, however, being retained. It is this marbleing that gives flavor and tenderness to the meat.

FACT: Growth Hormones Not Harmful to Humans.
Natural and synthetic growth hormone products are used to accelerate growth in beef animals. These products result in increased growth of lean muscle tissue in the animals, while doing away with fat. All products are approved by the Food and Drug Administration on the basis of very stringent tests for safety. There is no evidence of any human health problem from the use of any of these products.

*Facts were taken from **The Story of Modern Beef**, produced by the National Cattlemen's Association for the Beef Promotion and Research Board, © 1988.*

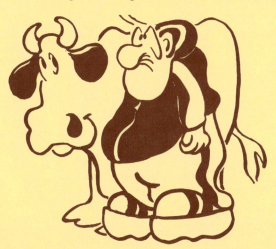

Remember...
Cooking beef
to at least 150 degrees, thawing frozen beef in the refrigerator, thoroughly washing hands, food utensils and all surfaces that come in contact with uncooked meat, storing leftovers immediately, and reheating leftovers thoroughly are safeguards against food contamination and poisoning.

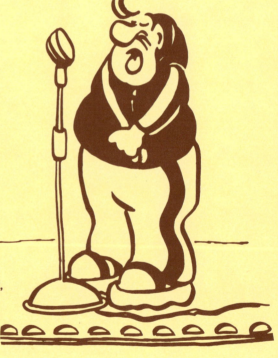

Beef, Wonderful Beef

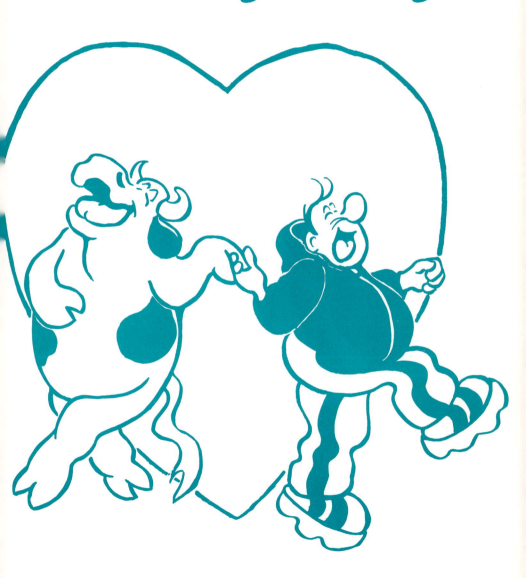

Preparing and Serving Beef

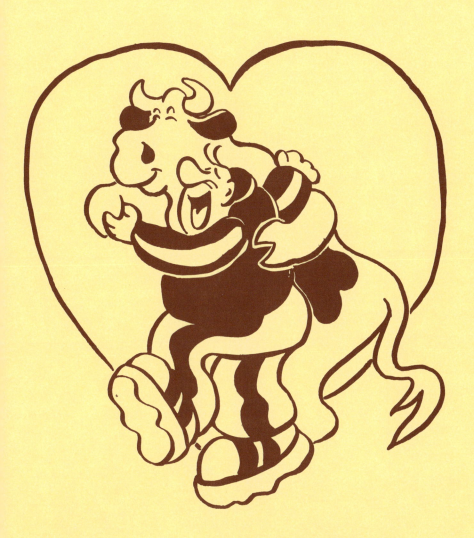

Cooking Beef	54	Beef Menus	
Microwave Tips	61	Beef Salads	73
Carving	64	Beef Soups	85
		Beef Stir-Fry	95
The Salad:	65	Beef Burgers &	
Beef's Perfect		Sandwiches	103
Complement		Beef Marinades	113
Ree Zaphiropoulos		Beef Main Entrees	119

Cooking Beef

It is important to choose the best method of cooking beef to produce flavorful, juicy, and tender beef dishes. The choice of cooking method depends on the cut of beef itself and the tenderness of the particular piece of beef. Tender cuts may be cooked by dry heat methods. Less tender cuts should be cooked by moist heat methods. The lower cooking temperature and the longer cooking time enables some less tender cuts to be cooked by dry heat methods. It is also possible to tenderize less tender cuts.

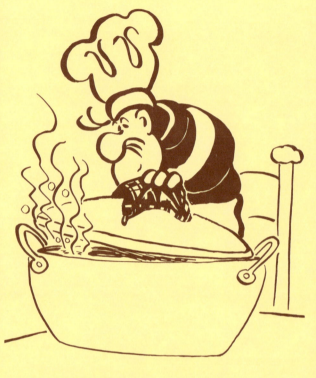

Tenderizing

Less tender cuts of meat can be just as tasty as the top cuts if some time is spent on tenderizing the cuts before cooking them. These cuts can then be cooked successfully by a dry heat method.

Pounding
Pounding with a heavy object such as a meat mallet tenderizes by breaking down the beef fibers, particularly the connective tissue.

Marinades

Marinades are liquids which traditionally contain some sort of food acid, such as vinegar, wine, lemon juice, other citrus juice or tomato juice. The acid helps soften the meat fibers and connective tissues. It also adds flavor. Most marinades also contain a small amount of oil and are especially appropriate for beef cuts which have little natural fat, but care should be taken in using any oil in regards to a low fat diet. Place beef in a marinade under refrigeration for 6 to 24 hours.

Dry Heat Methods

Roasting

Season meat, if desired. Place beef, fat side up, on a rack in an open pan. Insert meat thermometer (do not rest in fat or on the bone). Do not add water. Do not cover. Roast in slow oven, 300°F - 325°F. Roast to 5° below desired degree of doneness to allow for continued cooking after the removal from the oven.

Broiling

Place beef on rack in broiler pan 2 to 5 inches from heat. Broil until surface is browned. Season if desired. Turn meat and cook until done. Season second side.

Panbroiling

Place beef in preheated frying pan. Do not add oil or water. Do not cover. Cook slowly, turning occasionally, (5/8 to 1 inch cuts). Over medium heat. Pour off excess drippings as they accumulate. Season if desired.

Pan or Stir-Frying

Place beef in small amount of heated oil. Do not cover. Cook at medium temperature for pan frying and over high heat for stir-frying. Brown on both sides for pan frying. Turn meat pieces over continuously for stir-frying. Season as desired. Remove from pan and serve at once.

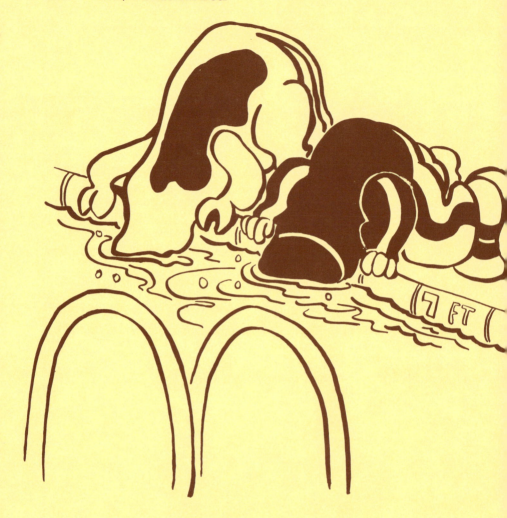

Moist Heat Methods

Braising
 Brown beef in small amount of oil in heavy skillet. Pour off drippings. Season if desired. Add small amount of liquid. Cover tightly. Cook at low temperature until tender.

Cooking in Liquid
 Coat beef with seasoned flour if desired. Brown on all sides in small amount of oil. Pour off excess drippings. Cover with liquid. Season if desired. Cover tightly and simmer until tender.

Cooking Tips

♥ **Choose the most appropriate cooking method to produce flavorful, tender, and juicy beef. Your choice depends on the cut and tenderness of the beef.**

♥ **Use only lean portions, trim all visible fat.**
The rule of thumb is that a 4-ounce portion of uncooked beef is a 3-ounce serving, and contains 8 grams of total fat and less than 3 grams of saturated fat, under 76 grams of cholesterol and is about 180 calories.

♥ **Marinate with herbs, garlic, wine, or lemon juice, not oil.**

♥ **Drain all cooked meat well. Skim fat off soups, sauces, and stews.**

♥ **Do not salt beef prior to cooking. Salt draws moisture from the meat and prevents browning.**

♥ **Cook beef to at least medium to maximize fat loss.**

Grilling Tips

♥ **Cook steaks hot and cook them fast.**

♥ **Select steaks that are at least one inch thick.**

♥ **Prepare coals until they are covered with ash.**

♥ **Place steaks 4 to 6 inches from coals.**

♥ **Place steaks to be cooked "well done" on the grill first.**

♥ **Grill until well browned, turn, season if desired. Grill the second side until the degree of cooking is achieved, and then season the second side.**

NOTE: Lean cuts, such as round and sirloin steaks are best cut thick and marinated prior to grilling for extra flavor and tenderness. Top loin and tenderloin steak can be enhanced by a zesty salsa.

Timetable for Broiling

Cut	Approximate Weight	Inches From Heat	Cooking Time (Min) Rare	Med.
Chuck Steak				
3/4 inch	1-1/4 to 1-3/4 pounds	2 to 3	14	20
1 inch	1-1/2 to 1-1/2 pounds	3 to 4	20	25
1-1/2 inches	2 to 4 pounds	4 to 5	30	35
Rib Steak				
3/4 inch	11 to 14 ounces	2 to 3	8	12
1 inch	1 to 1-1/2 pounds	3 to 4	15	20
1-1/2 inches	1-1/2 to 2 pounds	4 to 5	25	30
Rib Eye Steak				
3/4 inch	7 to 8 ounces	2 to 3	8	12
1 inch	9 to 10 ounces	3 to 4	14	20
1-1/2 inches	12 to 14 ounces	4 to 5	25	30
Top Loin Steak				
3/4 inch	11 to 14 ounces	2 to 3	8	12
1 inch	1 to 1-1/2 pounds	3 to 4	15	20
1-1/2 inches	1-1/2 to 2 pounds	4 to 5	25	30
Sirloin Steak				
3/4 inch	1-1/4 to 1-3/4 pounds	2 to 3	10	15
1 inch	1-1/2 to 3 pounds	3 to 4	20	25
1-1/2 inches	2-1/4 to 4 pounds	4 to 5	30	35
Porterhouse Steak				
3/4 inch	12 to 16 ounces	2 to 3	10	15
1 inch	1-1/2 to 2 pounds	3 to 4	20	25
1-1/2 inches	2 to 3 pounds	4 to 5	30	35
Tenderloin				
(Filet Mignon)	4 to 8 ounces	2 to 4	10-15	15-20
Ground Beef Patties				
1/2 inch x 4 inches	4 ounces	3 to 4	8	12
1 inch x 4 inches	5-1/3 ounces	3 to 4	12	18
Top Round Steak				
1 inch	1-1/4 to 1-3/4 pounds	3 to 4	20	30
1-1/2 inches	1-1/2 to 2 pounds	4 to 5	30	35
Flank Steak	1 to 1-1/2 pounds	2 to 3	12	14

Timetable for Roasting
(300°F to 325°F Oven Temperature)

Cut	Approx. Weight	Meat Thermometer Reading	Approx.* Total Cooking Time
	Pounds		Min. per lb.
Rib[1]	6 to 8	140°F(rare)	23 to 25
		160°F(medium)	27 to 30
		170°F (well)	32 to 35
Rib[1]	4 to 6	140°F (rare)	26 to 32
		160°F (medium)	34 to 38
		170°F(well)	40 to 42
Rib Eye[2] (Delmonico)	4 to 6	140°F(rare)	18 to 20
		160°F(medium)	20 to 22
		170°F(well)	22 to 24
Tenderloin Whole[3] (total)	4 to 6	140°F (rare)	45 to 60
Tenderloin Half[3] (total)	2 to 3	140°F (rare)	45 to 50
Boneless Rump	4 to 6	150°F-170°F	25 to 30
Tip	3-1/2 to 4	140°F-170°F	35 to 40
	6 to 8	140°F-170°F	30 to 35
Top Round	4 to 6	140°F-170°F	25 to 30
Ground Beef Loaf (9x5")	1-1/2 to 3-1/2	160°F -170°F	1 to 1-1/2 hrs

*Based on meat taken directly from refrigerator.
[1]Ribs which measure 6 to 7 inches from chine bone to tip of rib.
[2]Roast at 350°F oven temperature.
[3]Roast at 425°F oven temperature.

Timetable for Braising

Cut	Approximate Weight or Thickness	Approximate Total Cooking Time
Blade Pot Roast	3 to 5 pounds	2 to 2-1/2 hours
Arm Pot Roast	3 to 5 pounds	2-1/2 to 3-1/2 hours
Boneless Chuck Roast	3 to 5 pounds	2-1/2 to 3-1/2 hours
Short Ribs	Pieces (2 in. x 2 in. x 4 in.)	2-1/2 to 3-1/2 hours
Flank Steak	1-1/2 to 2 pounds	1-1/2 to 2-1/2 hours
Round Steak	3/4 to 1 inch	1 to 1-1/2 hours
Swiss Steak	1-1/2 to 2-1/2 inches	2 to 3 hours

Timetable for Cooking in Liquid

Cut	Approximate Weight	Approximate Total Cooking Time
Fresh or Corned Brisket	4 to 6 pounds	3-1/2 to 4-1/2 hours
Shank Cross Cuts	3/4 to 1-1/4 pounds	2-1/2 to 3 hours
Beef for Stew		2 to 3 hours

Tips for Cooking Beef in A Microwave Oven

♥ When cooking beef in a microwave, there is no need to add fats or oils to prevent sticking.

♥ Small pieces cook faster than large pieces, thin parts faster than thick parts, and small quantities faster than large quantities. So it is important to try to have similar sized pieces of beef placed evenly in the oven and to rotate pieces equally.

♥ Use a microwave-safe meat thermometer when cooking roasts. As in traditional beef cooking, remove the beef when the thermometer reads 5° below the desired degree of doneness. Cover the roast with foil and let stand 15 minutes before carving.

♥ Cook roast on a rack and cover with waxed paper to prevent splattering in your oven.

♥ Top round, top loin and round tip roast can all be cooked in a microwave oven. Select boneless, uniform roasts under 4 pounds. Always trim any visible fat. Microwave, fat side down, on medium low (30% power) about 20 minutes per pound. Roasts are most uniform in doneness throughout when cooked at a low power setting. Rotate to ensure even cooking.

♥ Top round and sirloin cut into cubes or strips are best microwaved using a moist heat method.

♥ Cook all beef cuts, except ground beef, on medium low (30%) to medium (50%) power to develop tenderness and flavor. Ground beef is already tenderized by the grinding process and can stand high power.

Beef, Wonderful Beef

♥ When cooking ground beef, drain the excess fat often, giving a final draining in a strainer or on a paper towel.

♥ Very nice microwave cooking pans are now available, including a pressure cooker especially designed for microwave use. By following the manufacturer's instructions, excellent results may be achieved.

♥ Above all, remember that timing is very important in a microwave oven. Be sure to consider the following factors when establishing cooking times:
- colder foods take longer to cook than those at room temperature.
- outer edges and thin, flat shapes cook more quickly.
- foods high in fat and sugar cook more quickly.
- high moisture foods cook more slowly.
- more food requires longer cooking time.
- larger pieces of food continue to cook when removed from the oven therefore it is best to slightly undercook the food and allow for standing time.

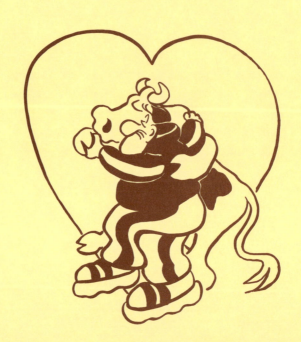

Beef, Wonderful Beef   63

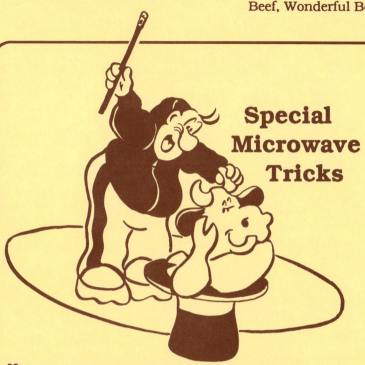

Special Microwave Tricks

♥ **To Remove Extra Fat from Ground Beef**
Crumble groud beef into a colander and place the colander over a dish in the microwave to catch the draining fat. Microwave on high power, stirring at least once.

♥ **To Enhance the Appearance of Beef**
• brush the surface of the meat with a dark liquid such as lite soy sauce or Worcestershire sauce.
• sprinkle the surface with gravy or soup mix.
• add a sauce or glaze, but remember those high in sugar will brown more readily.
• pre-brown the beef in a frying pan before cooking.
• use a microwave browning dish, following manufacturer's instructions.

♥ **To Enhance the Tenderness of Less Tender Cuts**
• Cook less tender meat cuts more slowly
• cover beef with plastic wrap or place in a cooking bag and extend the cooking time.
• use a simmer pot designed for a microwave oven.
• cook other foods such as rice or vegetable with the beef.
• marinate the beef in a liquid containing a food acid, such as vinegar or lemon juice, before cooking.
• pound or cut beef into thin strips.

Carving Beef

Proper carving makes meat seem more tender. You need a good, razor-sharp knife, a good cutting board and some knowledge of the meat to be carved.

Meat is made up of bundles of long muscle fibers held together with connective tissue. Fibers would be difficult or impossible to chew if they weren't made softer and shorter. Proper cooking softens the fibers and connective tissues. Proper carving shortens the fibers.

The direction in which the muscle fibers run is called the grain. The principle of meat carving is to cut across the grain. This is a simple principle, but carving itself is not always as simple. Some roasts are made up of more than one muscle, and the fibers in each of the different muscles may run in slightly different directions. This makes finding the grain more difficult.

Contrary to most carving rules, some tender steaks are carved with the grain. Steaks from the short loin and the sirloin need not be cut across the grain because the meat fibers are tender and already relatively short.

Steps to Carving

1. Remove the roast from the oven and let it sit for 15 to 20 minutes before carving so that it will be juicier and easier to serve. (If steaks are to be carved, do so immediately.)

2. Determine which way the muscle fibers run in the meat. This is the grain.

3. Anchor the meat firmly with a two-pronged carving fork.

4. Slice roasts across the grain. Carve tender steaks with the grain. Carve less tender steaks (such as top round or flank) diagonally across the grain into thin slices.

The Salad

Beef's Perfect Complement

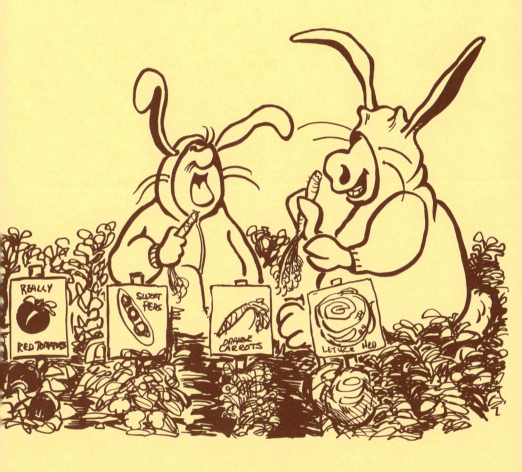

Basic Vinaigrette	68	Hearts of Palm Salad	70
Renn's "Red" Dressing	68	Hearts of Palm with	71
San Francisco Dinner Salad	69	Asparagus Salad	
		Fresh Beet Salad	71
Japanese Salad	69	Sliced Cucumber Salad	72
Green and White Salad	70	Three Color Salad	72

The Salad Philosophy
contributed by
Ree Zaphiropoulos

My daughter, Gale, inspired me to describe my salads in recipe form. There is no right or wrong way to make a salad. I was raised on oil and vinegar salads, and I learned by watching my Swiss grandmother pour oil and vinegar by eye— the only way as far as I am concerned. Our family still likes a tart salad and, to this day, that is my idea of a "real" salad.

Salad ingredients are always readily available. The fun of making a salad is the way you slice, chop, and mix the ingredients. Presentation can make the simplest salad a work of art. Anything fresh, crisp, and cold is good in a salad. Some of my best creations have come from cleaning out the refrigerator.

Suggestions and Observations

♥   Use Italian olive oil.

♥   Use unflavored red wine vinegar.

♥   Use only the freshest lettuce and vegetables.

♥   Use two or three types of lettuce in the same salad for variation.

♥   Use thinly sliced scallion, red yellow onions, or shallots in small amounts in the same salad.

♥   Use red, white, and Napa cabbage for added texture and color.

♥   Chop vegetables in different shapes.

♥   Lettuce and vegetables should be dry and cold before mixing.

♥   Always taste before serving - in doubt, add vinegar or a little salt.

Beef, Wonderful Beef

♥ Mix salad at the last minute to prevent wilting. Cut vegetables or lettuce in a size that is easy to eat.

♥ Mix dressing in a jar with a tight-fitting lid so you can shake it vigorously prior to adding to the salad. I like to use a Dijon mustard jar.

♥ Salads should be small when serving several courses.

♥ Salad too tart or salty? Add grated hard boiled egg and/or Parmesan cheese.

♥ Out of vinegar, use lemon juice.

♥ Out of Dijon mustard, use Coleman mustard.

♥ Use salted water when blanching vegetables.

♥ Run cold water over blanched or steamed vegetables so they stop cooking. Drain well, chill well.

♥ Purchase a garnishing kit. There are wonderful tools to make vegetable flowers, and other designs.

♥ Use all the different types of parsley, watercress, mint and other greens available for garni.

♥ Flowers are beautiful for garni. Use flowers of the season, such as holly or poinsettia for Christmas or lillies at Easter.

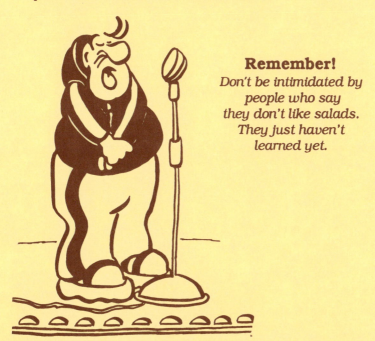

Remember!
Don't be intimidated by people who say they don't like salads. They just haven't learned yet.

Basic Vinaigrette

1/3 cup red wine vinegar
2/3 cup Italian olive oil
1 teaspoon salt
Fresh ground pepper

This is my basic tart vinaigrette. More oil can be added for a milder dressing, but please don't tell me.

Variations:
        Add 1 tablespoon Dijon mustard
        Add 1/4 teaspoon garlic
        Add 1/4 teaspoon fine herbs, oregano, dill, sweet basil
        Add 1 tablespoon Worcestershire sauce

serving, 1 tablespoon   0.0 milligrams cholesterol
per serving information   1.35 grams saturated fat
84 calories   9.50 grams fat

Renn's "Red" Dressing

1/4 cup vinegar
2 tablespoons catsup
1 teaspoon sweet basil
1/2 cup oil
1 teaspoon sugar
Dash of salt

Mix all ingredients in jar and shake well.

6 servings   0.0 milligrams cholesterol
per serving information   1.10 grams saturated fat
70 calories   7.71 grams fat

San Francisco Dinner Salad

1 head butter lettuce
1 slice cucumber per person
1/4 tomato per person
1 artichoke heart or 3 marinated mushrooms per person

Mix with herbed vinaigrette. Arrange salad on plate so that each person has lettuce plus the last three ingredients.

1 serving
per serving information
76 calories

0.0 milligrams cholesterol
.84 grams saturated fat
5.93 grams fat

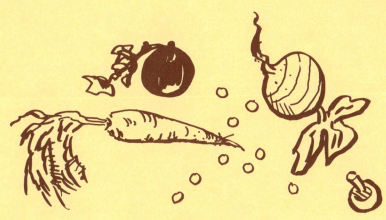

Japanese Salad

1/2 head of head lettuce
2 tablespoons water chestnuts, sliced
2 scallions, sliced
1/4 cup frozen or fresh peas, parboiled
1/3 cup small snow peas
6 radishes, sliced

Mix above ingredients in vinaigrette that has 2 tablespoon soy sauce and 1 teaspoon brown sugar added. Good, even if it isn't as tart as usual.

4 servings
per serving information
77 calories

0.0 milligrams cholesterol
1.03 grams saturated fat
7.25 grams fat

Green and White Salad

1/4 head white cabbage, thinly sliced
1/2 cup bean sprouts
1/2 cup snow peas, blanched
1 tablespoon parsley, chopped
1/2 yellow onion, sliced
1/2 cucumber, sliced
1/2 green pepper, sliced
1/4 bunch spinach leaves, cleaned
1/2 head Romaine lettuce
1/2 cup raw cauliflower, thinly sliced

Mix all the above ingredients with vinaigrette plus 1/4 cup light mayonaise. Salt and pepper to taste.

Note: Maui or Walla Walla onions are wonderful alternatives.

8 servings
per serving information
70 calories

2.5 milligrams cholesterol
0.538 grams saturated fat
5.75 grams fat

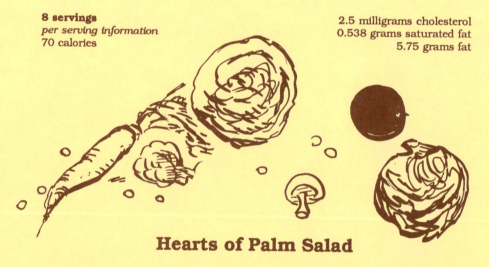

Hearts of Palm Salad

Slice hearts of palm lengthwise. Marinate in vinaigrette. Arrange on plates, 3 slices per serving. Place on top of large leaf of Boston lettuce. Put a little chipped egg in the middle of the hearts of palm. Add a tomato rose for color. Don't forget a sprig of parsley. A red bell pepper round is also pretty if you don't have time for the rose.

1 serving
per serving information
28 calories

0.0 milligrams cholesterol
.45 grams saturated fat
3.167 grams fat

Hearts of Palm with Asparagus

Marinate hearts of palm in vinaigrette. Blanch asparagus tips, rinse, cool, and marinate. Arrange on salad plate with or without large lettuce leaf.

Variations: Add chopped egg, shrimp, red pepper or tomato for color. Garnish with parsley

1 serving
per serving information
50 calories

0.0 milligrams cholesterol
.514 grams saturated fat
3.447 grams fat

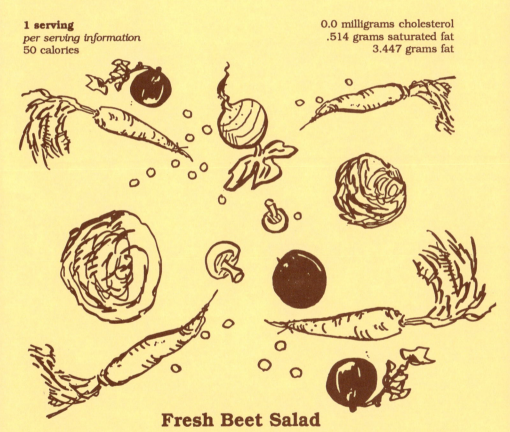

Fresh Beet Salad

Boil beets until al dente, cool. Slice Bermuda or torpedo onion in rings. Slice beets in 1/4-inch rounds, mix with onion rings, and marinate in vinaigrette. The longer they marinate the better.

serving, 1/2 cup
per serving information
45 calories

0.0 milligrams cholesterol
.327 grams saturated fat
2.29 grams fat

Sliced Cucumber Salad

Peel cucumbers and thinly slice Maui onions. Marinate in vinaigrette. Arrange in rings on individual serving dishes.

serving, per cup
per serving information
5 calories

0.0 milligrams cholesterol
.674 grams saturated fat
4.64 grams fat

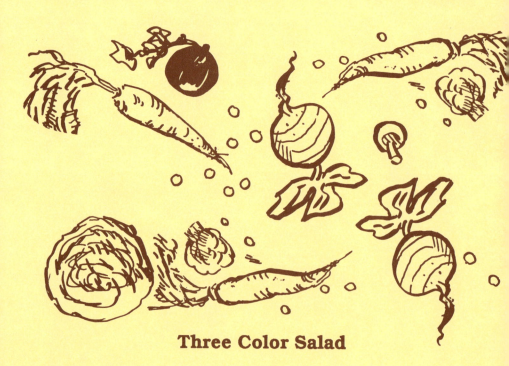

Three Color Salad

Blanch and cool
Snow peas
Cauliflowerets
Carrot rounds

Marinate in vinaigrette.

Variations: Chop red bell pepper for pretty color addition. Steam large shrimp and add for additional jazz.

serving, per cup
per serving information
66 calories

0.0 milligrams cholesterol
.656 grams saturated fat
4.65 grams fat

Beef Salads

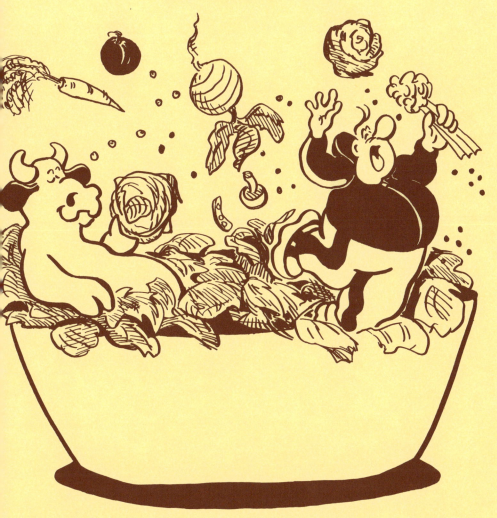

Beef and Asparagus Salad	74	Pasta Beef Salad	80
California Ground Sirloin Salad	75	Deluxe Steak Salad	81
		Beef and Dill Pickle Salad	82
Tomato Beef Salad	76		
Ross's Beef Salad	77	Lime Beef Salad	83
Marinated Beef Salad	78	Beef, Raspberry, and Kiwi Salad	84
Italian Beef Salad	79		

Beef and Asparagus Salad

1/3 cup lite soy sauce
1/4 cup rice vinegar
1 tablespoon sesame or olive oil
1 tablespoon fresh ginger, grated
1 cup asparagus, cut diagonally into 1-inch pieces
1 cup broccoli flowers
3/4 pound roast beef, thinly sliced
     cut into julienne strips
4 cups lettuce, shredded
1 cup mushrooms, thinly sliced
1 cup sweet red pepper, cut into thin strips
1 cup red onion, thinly sliced

Combine soy sauce, vinegar, oil, and ginger. In boiling water blanch asparagus and broccoli. Rinse in cold water and drain well. Toss the beef with 1/2 cup of the dressing. To serve, arrange greens, asparagus, broccoli, mushrooms, pepper, and onion on a platter. Place beef in center. Either serve the rest of the dressing on the side or drizzle it over the other ingredients.

6 servings
per serving information
200 calories
45.90 milligrams cholesterol
3.68 grams saturated fat
10.50 grams fat

California Ground Sirloin Salad

12 ounces top-grade, ground beef
1/2 cup onion, chopped
1/4 teaspoon garlic salt
1/8 teaspoon freshly ground pepper
1 16-ounce can refried beans with green chilies
1 4-ounce can green chilies, chopped
1/2 cup low-fat sharp cheddar cheese, shredded
4 cups lettuce, shredded
1 tomato, chopped
1 4-ounce can ripe olives, sliced

In large skillet, brown beef. Add onion and saute lightly. Add salt, pepper, and green chilies. Push to one side of skillet, and heat the refried beans thoroughly. Place 1/4 of the beans in the center of each individual dinner plate. Top with 1/4 of the meat mixture. Place the shredded lettuce in a circle around the "tostada." Top with tomatoes and cheese and garnish with olives.

4 servings
per serving information
390 calories
84 milligrams cholesterol
6.54 grams saturated fat
19.70 grams fat

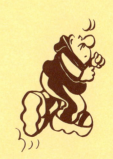

Tomato Beef Salad

8 fancy lettuce leaves
3 medium ripe tomatoes, cut in wedges
1 pound sirloin steak, cooked medium rare,
    sliced in 1/4-inch strips
8 mushrooms, thinly sliced
1 bunch green onions, thinly sliced
1 cup tart vinaigrette dressing
Fresh ground pepper to taste

Arrange 2 lettuce leaves on each individual salad plate. Alternate steak and tomatoes in circular design. Top with mushrooms and green onions. Spoon vinaigrette over salad. Season with pepper to taste. Garnish with parsley.

4 servings
per serving information
374.8 calories
75.94 milligrams cholesterol
7.165 grams saturated fat
26.42 grams fat

Ross's Beef Salad

12-15 small mushrooms, finely sliced
1 pound top sirloin, broiled or grilled, medium rare, carefully trimmed, sliced into thin strips
1 6-ounce jar artichoke hearts, drained, quartered
1 head iceberg lettuce, shredded
1 head purple/red lettuce
3 tablespoons blue cheese, crumbled (optional)

Combine the marinade and mix well. Add the cooked beef, the mushrooms, and artichokes. Refrigerate for 10 to 15 hours. To serve, arrange the iceberg lettuce on a bed of the red lettuce. Arrange the meat and vegetables on top of the lettuce. Pour marinade over meat mixture. Garnish with crumbled blue cheese.

4 servings
per serving information
192 calories
53.81 milligrams cholesterol
3.587 grams saturated fat
8.258 grams fat

Marinade
1/2 cup virgin olive oil
2 teaspoons Dijon mustard
2 cloves garlic, minced
Fresh ground pepper to taste

4 servings
per serving information
162 calories
0.0 milligrams cholesterol
2.559 grams saturated fat
18.12 grams fat

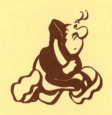

Marinated Beef Salad

8 fancy lettuce leaves
4 small limes
1 teaspoon fresh ginger, minced
2 teaspoons fresh parsley, chopped
1 teaspoon fresh mint, chopped
3 tablespoons olive oil
1 pound rare steak or roast beef, thinly sliced
8 mushrooms, thinly sliced
1 cantaloupe cut into balls
Freshly ground pepper to taste
Parsley and toasted sesame seeds for garnish

Squeeze enough fresh lime juice for 3 tablespoons. Grate lime peel to make 1 teaspoon. Cut remaining lime into thin slices for garnish. Combine lime juice, grated lime peel, ginger, parsley, mint, and olive oil for dressing.

Arrange 2 lettuce leaves on individual salad plates. Place steak in middle of leaves. Top with mushrooms. Arrange cantaloupe balls around edge. Spoon dressing over salad. Serve chilled. Garnish with freshly ground pepper, parsley, sesame seeds, and lime slice twists.

4 servings
per serving information
378.1 calories
75.94 milligrams cholesterol
5.591 grams saturated fat
20.92 grams fat

Italian Beef Salad

per salad
3 ounces roast beef, thinly sliced
1/2 ounce linguine noodles, cooked and chilled
10 snow peas, blanched and chilled
Red pepper sticks
Carrot slices
Zucchini slices
Red onion rings
Shredded lettuce
Tart vinaigrette

Arrange shredded lettuce on salad plate. Place noodles in center. Arrange vegetables and meat in spoke-like design around noodles. Pour dressing over noodles, meat, and vegetables. Garnish with parsley.

1 serving
per serving information
326.9 calories
80.37 milligrams cholesterol
5.652 grams saturated fat
18.49 grams fat

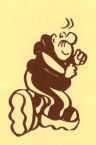

Pasta Beef Salad

4 ounces novelty macaroni
1 10-ounce package frozen broccoli
6 ounces well-trimmed roast beef, thinly sliced
1 6-ounce jar marinated artichoke hearts, drained
2 ripe tomatoes, cut into wedges
1 cup feta cheese, crumbled
1/2 cup low-calorie Italian salad dressing

Cook pasta according to package directions. Add broccoli
and boil for 3 minutes. Drain and rinse with cold ice water.
Cut beef into julienne strips. Quarter the artichokes. In a
large glass bowl, combine all ingredients. Refrigerate until
serving time. Serve well chilled.

4 servings
per serving information
271 calories
59.7 milligrams cholesterol
6.8 grams saturated fat
12.20 grams fat

Deluxe Steak Salad

1 1/2 pounds top sirloin steak all fat removed, grilled to medium rare, thinly sliced on the diagonal
1 4-ounce jar sliced mushrooms
1 green pepper, sliced into thin rings
1/3 cup red wine vinegar
1/4 cup olive oil
1/2 teaspoon garlic salt
1/2 teaspoon onion salt
1/2 teaspoon Worcestershire sauce
1 teaspoon freshly ground pepper
1/4 teaspoon tarragon
1/4 teaspoon basil
4 cups lettuce, shredded
8 cherry tomatoes, cut in half

Arrange the steak on the bottom of a 9x13" baking dish. Place mushrooms and peppers on top of steak. Combine vinegar, oil, and seasonings. Pour dressing over meat. Cover and refrigerate 5 to 6 hours. Drain well. Arrange steak and vegetables on lettuce bed and garnish with tomatoes. Serve with Dijon mustard or horseradish and parsley.

6 servings
per serving information
246 calories
67.3 milligrams cholesterol
4.533 grams saturated fat
15.10 grams fat

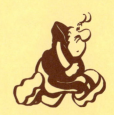

Beef and Dill Pickle Salad

8 fancy lettuce leaves
1 1/2 cups rare roast beef or steak, thinly sliced
1 cup celery, sliced diagonally
1/2 cup green onion, thinly sliced
1/4 cup green pepper, thinly sliced
1/4 cup red pepper, thinly sliced
1/2 cup dill pickle, quartered and thinly sliced

Dressing
1/2 cup olive oil
1/4 cup balsamic vinegar
1 tablespoon Dijon mustard
1 clove garlic, minced
Dash of Tabasco sauce
Freshly ground pepper

Combine all dressing ingredients and chill well. Arrange 2 lettuce leaves on each individual salad plate. Combine beef, celery, onion, peppers, and pickles. Toss. Place equal amount on lettuce leaves. Spoon dressing over salad. Garnish with freshly ground pepper, parsley, and cherry tomatoes.

4 servings
per serving information
129.8 calories
50.00 milligrams cholesterol
2.015 grams saturated fat
14.43 grams fat

Lime Beef Salad

1 pound sirloin steak, about 1-inch thick,
    well trimmed and grilled medium rare
2 large limes
1/4 cup lite soy sauce
1 teaspoon sugar
1 large sweet white onion, thinly sliced into rings
1 head bibb lettuce
8 mushrooms, thinly sliced
Fresh mint

Chill the steak, cut into thin diagonal slices. Save meat juices, removing any fat drippings.

Squeeze the juice from one lime (3 tablespoons). Cut other lime in 8 wedges for garnish. Combine lime juice, soy sauce, and sugar.

Arrange lettuce leaves on individual salad plates, place steak on top, and pour steak juice over meat. Place onion rings and mushrooms on top, with mint leaves on very top. Spoon sauce over all. Garnish with lime wedges.

6 servings
per serving information
170.1 calories
50.63 milligrams cholesterol
2.783 grams saturated fat
6.993 grams fat

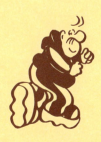

Beef, Raspberry, and Kiwi Salad

1 pound sirloin steak, medium rare, thinly sliced
1 head Belgium endive
1 head radicchio
1 cup raspberries
2 kiwis, peeled, thinly sliced
1/4 cup raspberry vinegar
7 teaspoons olive oil
Freshly ground pepper

Combine vinegar, olive oil, and pepper. Chill well.

Arrange endive and radicchio on individual serving plates. Place a circular ring of kiwi on lettuce. Place steak in center with raspberries around the edge. Spoon dressing over salad. Add additional freshly ground pepper to taste.

4 servings
per serving information
288 calories
75.94 milligrams cholesterol
4.785 grams saturated fat
15.01 grams fat

Beef Soups

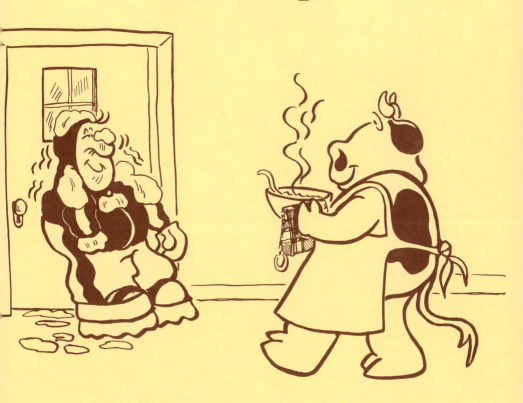

Oriental Style Hot and Sour Soup	86
Brandy Beef Soup	87
Beef Vegetable Rice Soup	88
Beef Barley Soup	89
"Camp-Out" Ground Beef Soup	90
Beef Vegetable Soup for a Crowd	91
Cajun Black Bean Soup	92
Spicy Red Bean Soup	93
Hearty Lentil Soup	94

Oriental Style Hot and Sour Soup

1 pound top sirloin, well trimmed,
    sliced 1/4-inch thick
1 cup lite soy sauce
4 cups water
1 tablespoon instant beef bouillon granules
8 mushrooms, thinly sliced
1 4-ounce can bamboo shoots, drained and julienned
1 cup bean sprouts
3 tablespoons red wine vinegar
1/4 teaspoon red pepper flakes
1/4 cup cold water
2 tablespoons cornstarch
1 egg, well beaten
1/4 cup green onions, thinly sliced

Pour soy sauce over beef slices. Bring water and bouillon granules to boil. Add beef, mushrooms, bamboo shoots, bean sprouts, vinegar, and pepper flakes. Simmer uncovered about 5 minutes. Combine water and cornstarch, slowly stir into soup and continue cooking until slightly thickened. Slowly pour egg into soup in a thin stream, stirring gently to make fine threads. Garnish with chopped green onions.

8 servings
per serving information
298.8 calories
144.4 milligrams cholesterol
4.584 grams saturated fat
11.76 grams fat

Brandy Beef Soup

2 pounds sirloin steak, well trimmed, cut into cubes
2 tablespoons margarine
2 tablespoons fresh orange peel, grated
12 boiling onions, peeled
3 cups double-strength beef broth
3/4 cup brandy
2 cloves garlic, minced
2 cups carrots, thinly sliced
2 tablespoons fresh lemon peel, grated
2 tablespoons fresh parsley, chopped
Freshly ground pepper

In a large soup kettle, melt margarine, and brown beef. Add orange peel and onions on top of meat. *Do not stir.* Add broth, 1/4 cup of brandy, and garlic. Cover and simmer at very low temperature for 3 hours. *Do not stir.* Add carrots. Cover and simmer for 1/2 hour. Add the remaining ingredients. Heat thoroughly. Add additional water if soup is too thick. Garnish with chopped parsley.

10 servings
per serving information
226 calories
60.87 milligrams cholesterol
3.577 grams saturated fat
9.490 grams fat

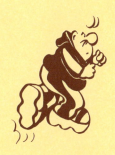

Beef Vegetable Rice Soup

3 cups beef broth
1/2 cup white onion, chopped
1 cup green pepper, cut in strips
1/2 cup celery, cut diagonally
2 10-ounce packages frozen mixed vegetables
1 16-ounce can whole tomatoes
1/4 cup brown rice, uncooked
3 cups beef, cut into cubes
1 clove garlic, minced
1 teaspoon Italian seasoning
Salt and pepper to taste
1 cup white wine

Heat broth to boil. Add all other ingredients except the wine. Cover and simmer until vegetables are tender. Add additional water if soup is too thick. Add wine before serving.

8 servings
per serving information
278 calories
50.9 milligrams cholesterol
2.9 grams saturated fat
7.32 grams fat

Beef Barley Soup

2 quarts water
1 large beef soup bone with meat
1/2 cup celery tops, chopped
1 tablespoon salt
1 teaspoon freshly ground pepper
1/2 cup raw barley
3 cups cabbage, chopped (1/2 green and 1/2 red is colorful)
1 large white onion, chopped
1 1/2 cups celery, diagonally sliced
1 1/2 cups carrots, sliced
1 12-ounce can tomato paste

In a large soup pot, combine first five ingredients. Bring to boil. Cover and simmer 2 to 3 hours. Remove bone from broth. Remove meat from bone and cut into small, bite-sized pieces. Add meat and barley to broth. Simmer 45 minutes. Add remaining ingredients and simmer until vegetables are tender, about 45 minutes.

12 servings
per serving information
206.5 calories
50.63 milligrams cholesterol
2.814 grams saturated fat
7.172 grams fat

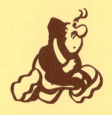

"Camp-Out" Ground Beef Soup

1 pound ground lean beef
1 cup potatoes, chopped
1 cup celery, sliced diagonally
1 cup carrots, sliced
1 cup white onions, chopped
1 large can whole tomatoes, coarsely chopped
4 cups water
2 teaspoons garlic salt
1 teaspoon fresh ground pepper
1/2 teaspoon Italian seasoning
1 cup cooked pasta, macaroni, or specialty noodles

Brown beef and drain well. Add vegetables, water, and seasonings. Cover and simmer 45 minutes until vegetables are tender. Add pasta shortly before serving. Garnish with finely chopped white onions.

6 servings
per serving information
160 calories
42 milligrams cholesterol
1.15 grams saturated fat
3.38 grams fat

Beef Vegetable Soup for a Crowd

1 20-ounce can tomatoes
6 cups water
2 pounds boneless chuck, cut in 1-inch cubes
2 teaspoons salt
1 teaspoon freshly ground pepper
1 cup celery, sliced
1/4 cup parsley, chopped
1/2 cup barley
2 16-ounce cans V-8™ juice
1 10-ounce package frozen beans
2 cups carrots, sliced
2 cups onions, chopped
1 teaspoon Worcestershire sauce
2 beef bouillon cubes

Combine all ingredients. Bring to boil, then simmer for 1 to 2 hours, uncovered. Add additional water if soup is too thick.

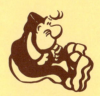

14 servings
per serving information
180 calories
36 milligrams cholesterol
2.64 grams saturated fat
6.42 grams fat

Cajun Black Bean Soup

1 pound dry black beans
1 1/2 pounds top grade sirloin, well trimmed,
    cut into cubes
1 1/2 quarts water
1/2 cup onion, minced
1 teaspoon cayenne pepper
2-3 tablespoons chili powder
1/2 teaspoon cumin
1 teaspoon salt
1/2 cup chili peppers, chopped

Combine beans, beef, and water in a large kettle. Heat to boiling. Reduce heat and simmer 2 to 3 hours. Stir frequently. Add other ingredients when bean skins pop open to indicate that they are cooked (sometimes you have to remove them from the pot and blow on them). Cover pot and simmer up to 2 hours. Remove 1/2 the soup and puree. Return puree to soup pot. Add more water if the mixture is too thick. This soup improves in flavor, extra good the day after it is made.

10 servings
per serving information
172 calories
40.48 milligrams cholesterol
2.64 grams saturated fat
5.64 grams fat

Spicy Red Bean Soup

1 teaspoon cayenne pepper
1 teaspoon fresh ground pepper
2 bay leaves
1 teaspoon ground cumin
1 pound dry red kidney beans
3 quarts water
1 pound sirloin steak, well trimmed,
    cut into cubes
1/2 teaspoon salt
1 1/2 cups celery, chopped
1 1/2 cups onion, chopped
3 cloves garlic, minced
Tabasco sauce to taste

Rinse beans and place all ingredients in a large soup kettle. Heat to boiling, reduce and simmer for 3 to 5 hours, stirring occasionally. Be sure beans are tender. This soup is much better the day after it is made.

8 servings
per serving information
159 calories
34.8 milligrams cholesterol
1.91 grams saturated fat
4.95 grams fat

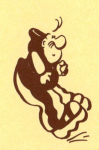

Hearty Lentil Soup

2 tablespoons olive oil
1 pound sirloin steak, well trimmed,
     cut into cubes
1 large white onion, chopped
3 stalks celery, chopped
2 cloves garlic, minced
1 cup lentils, rinsed
6 cups beef stock
1 large carrot, shredded
1 large potato, diced
1 16-ounce can tomatoes, chopped
1 cup red wine
Salt and freshly ground pepper to taste
Vinegar to taste

In large soup kettle, brown steak, saute onion, celery, and
garlic in oil until slightly browned, adding stock if needed.
Add lentils, stock, vegetables, and wine. Add salt and
pepper. Cover tightly and simmer 3 hours or until lentils
are tender. Adding vinegar into individual servings, 1
tablespoon at a time, is a nice change in taste. Garnish
with fresh parsley.

8 servings
per serving information
227.3 calories
37.97 milligrams cholesterol
2.573 grams saturated fat
8.611 grams fat

Beef Stir-Fry

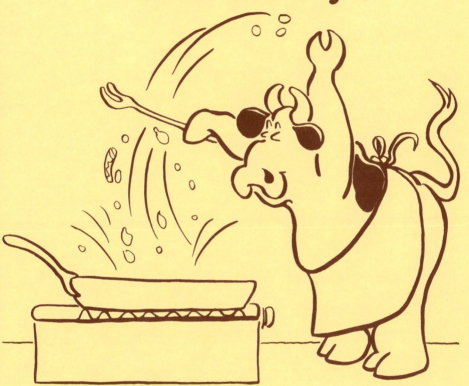

Chinese Beef and Rice	96
Beef with Cashews	97
Szechuan Beef with Peanuts	98
Tomato Beef	99
Spicy Broccoli Beef	100
Stir-Fry Orange Beef	101
Spicy Beef and Noodles	102

Chinese Beef and Rice

1 1/3 cups white rice, uncooked
2 tablespoons olive oil
1 teaspoon garlic salt
3 cups boiling water
2 beef bouillon cubes
2 tablespoons lite soy sauce
2 medium white onions, chopped
4 stalks celery, sliced on the diagonal
2 green peppers, cut into strips
3 cups well-trimmed lean beef, previoulsy cooked

In large skillet or wok, cook and stir rice in olive oil over medium heat until it is golden brown. Add salt, water, bouillon cubes, and soy sauce. Cover and simmer 20 minutes. Stir in onion, celery, green pepper, and meat. Cover and simmer 10 minutes longer or until all liquid is absorbed and rice is tender.

6 servings
per serving information
365 calories
101 milligrams cholesterol
5.21 grams. saturated fat
16.40 grams fat

Beef with Cashews

1 pound steak, well trimmed
4 tablespoon olive oil
10 mushrooms, sliced
10 green onions, chopped into 1/2-inch pieces
2 cloves garlic, minced
1 piece of fresh ginger, finely chopped
3/4 cup of unsalted cashews
1 cup water
2 tablespoons cornstarch
4 teaspoons lite soy sauce
1 cup peas
1/2 cup water chestnuts, sliced

Freeze meat slightly so that it is easy to slice thinly. Heat 2 tablespoons of the oil in skillet or wok at high heat. Stir-fry meat in oil until brown, 3 to 5 minutes. Remove. Heat remaining oil at high heat. Add onions, garlic, ginger, and cashews. Stir-fry 1 minute. Add meat to vegetable mixture. Combine all remaining ingredients and pour over meat mixture. Cook and stir until liquid boils and thickens. Serve with white rice.

6 servings
per serving information
338.9 calories
50.63 milligrams cholesterol
4.98 grams saturated fat
19.4 grams fat

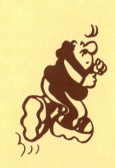

Szechuan Beef with Peanuts

1 tablespoon olive oil
1 slice fresh ginger, minced
1 clove garlic, minced
2 green onions, chopped
1 small dried hot chili pepper, minced
1 pound sirloin steak, well trimmed,
        cut into bite-sized pieces
1/2 cup unsalted peanuts
10 large fresh mushrooms, sliced
8 ounces fresh snow peas (broccoli may be substituted)
1 cup beef stock
2 tablespoons soy sauce
2 tablespoons sherry
1 tablespoon cornstarch
3 tablespoons cold water

Heat oil in wok or large skillet. Add next 4 ingredients and cook over high heat 2 minutes. Add beef and saute 2 to 4 minutes (until just cooked through). Add nuts, mushrooms, and vegetables and continue cooking 3 to 4 minutes, stirring constantly. Combine stock, soy sauce, and sherry. Add to the beef mixture. Heat through. Combine cornstarch and water and add to wok. Stir as mixture thickens.

4 servings
per serving information
393 calories
77 milligrams cholesterol
5.9 grams saturated fat
22.80 grams fat

Tomato Beef

1 pound top sirloin steak, well trimmed,
    cut into thin strips
2 tablespoons cornstarch
3 tablespoons sherry
1 tablespoon lite soy sauce
1 tablespoon olive oil
1 white onion, halved and cut into thin rings
4 cloves garlic, minced
4 ripe tomatoes, cut into quarters
1/2 cup green onions, thinly sliced

Combine cornstarch, sherry, and soy sauce. Add beef, toss well, cover, and refrigerate 1/2 hour. Heat a heavy skillet, add oil, and brown beef slightly. Add onion and garlic and saute for 3 minutes. Add tomatoes and continue cooking until thoroughly heated. Serve with white rice. Garnish with green onions.

6 servings
per serving information
205 calories
50.63 milligrams cholesterol
3.106 grams saturated fat
9.246 grams fat

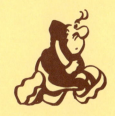

Spicy Broccoli Beef

1 tablespoon olive oil
1 pound top sirloin steak, well trimmed, thinly sliced
3 cups broccoli
1/2 cup water
1 teaspoon red pepper flakes
2 cloves garlic, minced
1/2 teaspoon ground ginger
1 1/2 teaspoons cornstarch
2 tablespoons lite soy sauce
1/4 cup low-calorie catsup
1/2 cup green onions, finely sliced

Heat oil in a heavy skillet, brown steak in oil. Remove steak from the skillet. Add broccoli, water, red pepper flakes, and garlic. Cover and steam for 5 minutes. Combine ginger, cornstarch, soy sauce, and catsup. Mix well. Return meat to skillet. Add cornstarch mixture. Bring to boil and continue cooking until sauce thickens. Serve with white rice and carrot sticks. Garnish with green onions.

6 servings
per serving information
184.9 calories
50.63 milligrams cholesterol
3.092 grams saturated fat
9.146 grams fat

Stir-Fry Orange Beef

1 pound sirloin steak, well trimmed, thinly sliced
2 egg whites
3 tablespoons cornstarch
1/2 cup sherry
3 tablespoons lite soy sauce
1/4 cup sugar
1/4 cup rice vinegar
1 tablespoon vegetable oil
1 tablespoon sesame oil
1 green pepper, cut in chunks
1/2 cup green onions, thinly sliced
1 zucchini, thinly sliced
3 tablespoons orange peel, grated

Beat egg whites until fluffy. Add next 5 ingredients and combine well. Add beef and toss. Marinate beef for 30 minutes. Drain beef, reserving marinade. Heat vegetable oil in heavy skillet. Brown beef, preventing pieces from sticking together. Remove beef from skillet and drain well. In skillet, heat sesame oil, add vegetables and orange peel. Stir-fry 2 minutes. Add meat and reserved marinade. Cook, stirring constantly, until thickened. Serve over rice. Garnish with parsley.

6 servings
per serving information
260.6 calories
50.63 milligrams cholesterol
3.719 grams saturated fat
13.59 grams fat

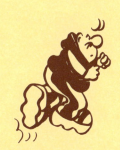

Spicy Beef and Noodles

1 pound sirloin steak, well trimmed, thinly sliced
4 tablespoons lite soy sauce
2 tablespoons cornstarch
3 tablespoons vegetable oil
3 tablespoons fresh ginger, grated
1/2 teaspoon sugar
2 cups hot water
8 ounces snow peas
1 cup bok choy, shredded
1 cup fresh bean sprouts
1 3-ounce package instant oriental noodles,
    including seasoning packet

Combine soy sauce and cornstarch. Add oil, ginger, and sugar. Blend well. Add beef. Toss. Marinate 1 hour. Bring water to boil, add remaining ingredients. Cook 3 to 4 minutes. Stir-fry beef in heavy skillet 2 to 3 minutes.

To serve, place beef on bed of noodles with vegetables. Garnish with parsley.

6 servings
per serving information
243.3 calories
50.63 milligrams cholesterol
3.637 grams saturated fat
14.15 grams fat

Beef Burgers and Sandwiches

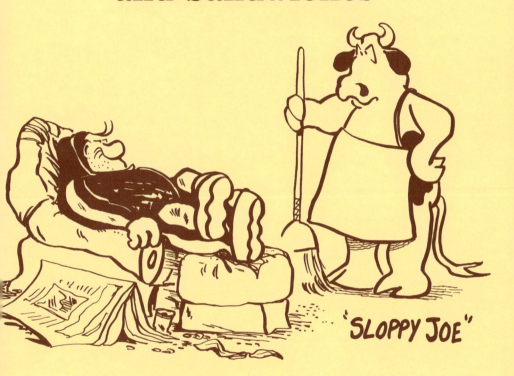

The Versatile Burger	104
Super French Burgers	105
Ortega Chili Burgers	106
Louisiana Burgers	107
Deluxe New Orleans Burgers	108
Low-Calorie Sloppy Joes	109
The Best Beef Sandwich You'll Ever Have	110
Florentine Beef Pita Bread Sandwiches	111
Open-Faced Beef Sandwiches	112

The Versatile Burger

1 1/2 pounds ground beef, lean
1/4 cup green pepper, finely chopped
1 medium white onion, finely chopped
1 stalk celery, finely chopped
1/4 teaspoon salt
1/2 teaspoon freshly ground pepper
1 large ripe beefsteak tomato, cut in 1/3-inch slices

Combine all ingredients except tomato. Shape into 6 patties. Broil 3 inches from heat about 4 to 5 minutes each side.

To serve, top each patty with tomato slice and garnish with parsley.

6 servings
per serving information
217 calories
67.10 milligrams cholesterol
5.17 grams saturated fat
13.30 grams fat

Super French Burgers

1 pound ground beef, lean
1/4 cup red wine
1 teaspoon thyme
1/4 cup green onions, thinly sliced
1 cup mushrooms, thinly sliced
1 cup white onions, chopped
3 tablespoons wine
Shredded lettuce

Combine beef, wine, thyme, and green onions. Shape into 6 patties. Broil or grill. Saute onions and mushrooms in wine.

To serve, place patties on shredded lettuce and top with sauteed mushrooms and onions. Garnish with parsley.

6 servings
per serving information
156 calories
50.63 milligrams cholesterol
2.764 grams saturated fat
6.846 grams fat

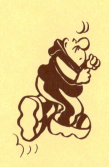

Ortega Chili Burgers

1 pound ground beef, lean
1/2 cup green onions, finely sliced
1 teaspoons Mrs. Dash™ seasoning
2 cloves garlic, minced
1 teaspoon cilantro
2 teaspoons from a package of Taco seasoning
1 8-ounce can chopped chilies
1 cup white onion, finely chopped
6 tablespoons salsa
Shredded lettuce

Combine beef, green onions, and seasonings. Shape into 6 patties. Broil or grill. Heat green chilies separately.

To serve, place meat on shredded lettuce and cover with heated chilies. Top with white onions and 1 tablespoon salsa. Garnish with parsley.

6 servings
per serving information
164.2 calories
50.63 milligrams cholesterol
2.764 grams saturated fat
7.205 grams fat

Louisiana Burgers

1 pound ground beef, lean
1 egg, lightly beaten
1/4 cup bread crumbs
1 tablespoon Cajun spices
4 slices white onion
4 slices tomato
4 crisp lettuce leaves

Combine egg, bread crumbs, and Cajun spices. Add meat and combine thoroughly. Shape into 4 patties. Broil or grill 4 to 6 minutes per side for medium rare.

To serve, place meat patties on lettuce leaf with onion and tomato slices on top. Garnish with parsley.

4 servings
per serving information
295 calories
143 milligrams cholesterol
7.47 grams saturated fat
19.60 grams fat

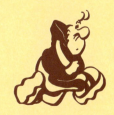

Deluxe New Orleans Burgers

1 pound ground beef, lean
1/2 cup green onions, thinly sliced
1 teaspoon Mrs. Dash™ seasoning
2 cloves garlic, minced
1 teaspoon basil
1 teaspoon parsley, chopped
1/2 teaspoon thyme
1/2 teaspoon Tabasco sauce
2 large white onions, thinly sliced in rings
1/4 cup white wine
Shredded lettuce

Combine all ingredients except onion rings and wine. Shape into 6 patties. Broil or grill. Saute white onion rings in wine.

To serve, place meat on shredded lettuce and cover with sauteed onions. Cherry tomatoes make a nice garnish.

6 servings
per serving information
161.5 calories
50.63 milligrams cholesterol
2.769 grams saturated fat
6.864 grams fat

Low-Calorie Sloppy Joes

1 pound ground beef, lean
1 large onion, chopped
2 cloves garlic, minced
1 6-ounce can Italian tomato paste
1/4 cup tomato or V-8™ juice
2 tablespoons Worcestershire sauce
1 tablespoon Dijon mustard
1 tablespoon lime juice
Freshly ground pepper
3 hamburger buns, split and toasted

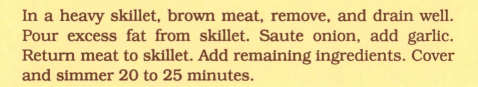

In a heavy skillet, brown meat, remove, and drain well. Pour excess fat from skillet. Saute onion, add garlic. Return meat to skillet. Add remaining ingredients. Cover and simmer 20 to 25 minutes.

To serve, divide meat mixture evenly over bun halves. Garnish with cherry tomatoes and parsley.

6 servings
per serving
234.6 calories
50.63 milligrams cholesterol
3.043 grams saturated fat
8.260 grams fat

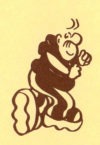

The Best Beef Sandwich
You'll Ever Have

8 slices low-calorie, whole wheat bread
1/2 pounds "deli" roast beef, thinly sliced
4 ounces low-calorie Swiss cheese, thinly sliced
1 4-ounce can chopped green chilies
Freshly ground pepper
4 tablespoons margarine

Assemble the sandwiches by evenly dividing the ingredients. Spread the margarine on the outside of the bread. Grill until golden, turning once.

4 servings
per serving information
321.9 calories
66.90 milligrams cholesterol
6.264 grams saturated fat
17.31 grams fat

Florentine Beef Pita Bread Sandwiches

4 whole wheat pita breads, cut in half
1/2 pound ground beef, lean
1 10-ounce package frozen spinach, chopped
1/2 pound mushrooms, thinly sliced
1/2 cup white onion, finely chopped
1/2 cup carrots, grated
2 cloves garlic, minced
1 teaspoons Mrs. Dash™ seasoning
1/2 teaspoon dill weed (optional)

Thaw frozen spinach and drain well. In a skillet, brown beef, remove, and drain well. In the same skillet, saute the onions and mushrooms, add other ingredients except pita bread. Combine well. Cook for 3 minutes, add beef and heat thoroughly. Warm pita breads, fill with mixture. Serve immediately.

8 servings
per serving information
127.6 calories
18.98 milligrams cholesterol
1.064 grams saturated fat
3.042 grams fat

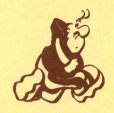

Open-Faced Beef Sandwiches

4 slices low-calorie, whole wheat bread
1/2 pound roast beef, thinly sliced
1/4 cup sweet onion, thinly sliced
Shredded lettuce
1 cup plain low-fat yogurt
1 tablespoon horseradish
1/4 teaspoon dill weed
1 teaspoon Dijon mustard
2 tablespoons green onions, very thinly sliced
Freshly ground pepper

Combine yogurt, horseradish, dill weed, mustard, green onions, and pepper. Mix well. Chill.

To serve, arrange lettuce and onion on bread, placing beef on top. Spoon sauce over each sandwich. Garnish with parsley or cherry tomatoes.

4 servings
per serving information
175.5 calories
38.97 milligrams cholesterol
2.181 grams saturated fat
5.793 grams fat

Beef Marinades

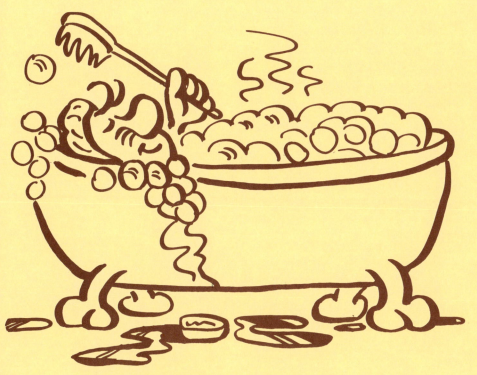

Great Beef Marinade — 114
Another Great Beef Marinade — 115
Burgundy Marinade — 116
Hawaiian Marinade — 116
Sesame Lime Marinade — 117

Great Beef Marinade

4 cloves garlic, crushed
1/4 cup olive oil
1 teaspoon rosemary
1 teaspoon oregano
1 teaspoon Dijon mustard
1 teaspoon lite soy sauce
1/4 cup tarragon vinegar
1/4 cup sherry

Shake all ingredients in a tightly-sealed jar. Marinate beef for at least 6 hours in a covered container.

serving, 1 tablespoon
per serving information
46 calories
0.0 milligrams cholesterol
.595 grams saturated fat
4.21 grams fat

Another Great Beef Marinade

1 teaspoon sugar
1 teaspoon garlic salt
1/2 teaspoon rosemary
1/2 teaspoons dry mustard
1/4 teaspoon ginger
1-2 teaspoon freshly ground pepper
2 tablespoons onion, minced
1/4 cup fresh lemon juice
1/3 cup olive oil
3 cloves garlic, minced
1/4 cup lite soy sauce
3 tablespoons honey
2 tablespoons vinegar

Place all ingredients in blender and blend until smooth. Marinate beef for at least 6 hours in a covered container.

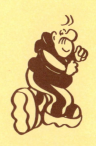

serving, 1 tablespoon
per serving information
44 calories
0.0 milligrams cholesterol
.483 grams saturated fat
3.40 grams fat

Burgundy Marinade

1 cup red wine
1 teaspoon Worcestershire sauce
1 tablespoon lite soy sauce
1/2 teaspoon oregano
1/2 teaspoon ground pepper

Combine all ingredients. Marinate beef for at least 6 hours in a covered container.

serving, 1 tablespoon
per serving information
10.44 calories
0.0 milligram cholesterol
0.002 grams saturated fat
0.006 grams fat

Hawaiian Marinade
(Great for Kabobs)

1 cup unsweetened pineapple juice
1/2 cup lite soy sauce
3 cloves garlic, crushed
1 teaspoon ginger
1/3 cup low-calorie Italian dressing

Combine all ingredients. Marinate beef for at least 6 hours in a covered container.

yield, 2 cups
serving, 1 tablespoon
per serving information
10.26 calories
0.165 milligrams cholesterol
0 035 grams saturated fat
0.259 grams fat

Sesame Lime Marinade

2/3 cup fresh lime juice
1/3 cup toasted sesame seeds
1 tablespoon lite soy sauce
1/3 cup low-calorie Italian dressing

Combine all ingredients. Marinate beef for at least 3 hours in a covered container.

serving, 1 tablespoon
per serving information
18.65 calories
0.240 milligrams cholesterol
0.199 grams saturated fat
1.440 grams fat

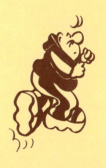

Remember...
Remain in control.
That is the most important rule. Remember, it is your body and your own good health.

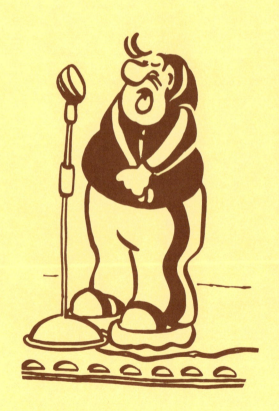

Main Courses

Steak

Chateaubriand	120
Sweet and Sour Grilled Steak	121
Dilly Steak	122
Salsa Marinated Steak	124

Roasts and Other Large Portions

Southwestern Style Beef Roast	125
Beef Brisket	126
New England Boiled Dinner	127

Barbeque and Ribs

Mustard Barbequed Roast Beef	128
Beef Brisket Barbeque	129
Our Favorite Beef Ribs	130
Oriental Garlic Short Ribs	131

Stews

Low-Fat Beef Stroganoff	132
Beer and Beef Stew	133
Burgundy Beef	134
Red Wine Sirloin Skillet	135

Ground, Stripped, and Cubed Beef

Fajitas	136
Marcos Mexican Steak Tartar	137
Simple Spaghetti Sauce	138
Thick Meat Sauce	139
Porcupines	140
Spanish Rice with Meat	141
Texas Skillet Supper	142
Curried Sweet Potato and Beef	143
Stuffed Green Peppers	144
Beef Stuffed Tomatoes	145
Shepherd's Pie	146
Hungarian Goulash	147
Sunday Morning Hash	148

Chateaubriand

2 pounds Chateaubriand
1 tablespoon Worcestershire sauce
1 tablespoon red wine vinegar
2 tablespoons brandy
1 tablespoon low-calorie catsup
4 cloves garlic, minced
1 teaspoon onion powder
Freshly ground pepper

Preheat oven to 450°F.

Place meat in roasting pan. Combine remaining ingredients. Spoon over meat. Marinate 1 to 2 hours. Insert meat thermometer and roast to medium rare. Be sure to check the thermometer often as the meat cooks quickly.

To serve, slice thinly and serve with fresh steamed vegetables. Garnish with parsley.

8 servings
per serving information
215.1 calories
75.94 milligrams cholesterol
4.117 grams saturated fat
10.08 grams fat

Sweet and Sour Grilled Steak

1 pound top sirloin steak, well trimmed
1/3 cup cider vinegar
1/4 cup honey
1/4 cup lite soy sauce
2 cloves garlic, minced
1/8 teaspoon Tabasco sauce

Combine all ingredients except steak in small saucepan. Cook over medium heat until honey is melted, about 5 minutes. Blend well and cook 1 minute more. Remove from heat. Pour cooled marinade over the steak. Refrigerate 6 to 18 hours. Turn every few hours. Drain steak. Reserve marinade. Grill steak, turning once. Baste with marinade often. Heat remaining marinade.

To serve, slice steak diagonally. Garnish with parsley. Serve heated marinade on the side.

6 servings
per service information
186.7 calories
50.63 milligrams cholesterol
2.745 grams saturated fat
6.720 grams fat

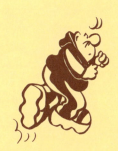

Dilly Steak

2 tablespoons flour
1/4 teaspoon salt
1/2 teaspoon freshly ground pepper
1 1/2 pounds sirloin steak, about 1/2-inch thick,
      well trimmed
1 tablespoon olive oil
1/2 cup water
3 tablespoons vinegar
1/2 teaspoon dried dill weed
2 large potatoes, peeled and sliced
2 medium zucchini, cut into 1 1/2-inch pieces
1/4 cup cold water
2 tablespoons flour
1/2 cup plain low-fat yogurt

Mix flour, salt, and pepper. Sprinkle one side of the beef with half the mixture and pound in. Turn meat and pound in remaining mixture. Cut beef into 6 equal pieces. Heat oil in large skillet. Cook beef over medium heat until brown, about 15 minutes. Mix 1/2 cup water, vinegar, and dill. Pour over beef. Heat to boiling and then reduce heat. Cover and simmer about 45 minutes or until beef is tender.

Add potatoes, cover and simmer 30 minutes. Add zucchini, cover and simmer 15 minutes. Remove beef and vegetables. Add enough water to make one cup liquid. Combine 1/4 cup water and flour. Gradually stir into broth. Heat to boiling, stirring constantly. Boil 1 minute and then stir in yogurt. Heat until hot and pour over beef and vegetables.

6 servings
per serving information
293 calories
76.3 milligrams cholesterol
4.49 grams saturated fat
12.50 grams fat

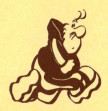

Salsa Marinated Steak

1 pound sirloin steak
1/2 cup salsa (medium or hot)
1/3 cup fresh lime juice
2 tablespoons hoisin* sauce
2 cloves garlic, minced

Combine salsa, lime juice, hoisin sauce, and garlic. Place steak in glass pan. Pour marinade over meat. Cover and refrigerate 6 to 8 hours, turning occasionally. Drain steak, reserving marinade. Broil or grill, brushing often with marinade, 14 minutes for rare, 18 minutes for medium.

To serve, slice thinly, garnish with parsley and cherry tomatoes.

* Available in the oriental spice section of your supermarket.

4 servings

per serving information
219 calories
75.94 milligrams cholesterol
4.12 grams saturated fat
10.80 grams fat

Southwestern Style Beef Roast

3 pounds beef eye-of-round roast
1/3 cup lite soy sauce
1/3 cup sherry
1/3 cup fresh lime juice
2 tablespoons olive oil
1 tablespoon fresh ginger, minced
1 tablespoon honey
4 cloves garlic, minced

Preheat oven to 325°F.

Combine all ingredients except beef. Place beef in glass pan. Pour marinade over meat. Cover and refrigerate at least 8 hours. Turn frequently. Remove roast, reserve marinade. Place roast on rack in uncovered roaster. Insert meat thermometer. Roast until thermometer reads 135° (20 to 22 minutes per pound). Brush roast with marinade during last 20 minutes of cooking. Heat remaining marinade. To serve slice roast thinly, drizzle heated marinade over meat.

8 servings
per serving information
214.8 calories
68.79 milligrams cholesterol
2.332 grams saturated fat
8.702 grams fat

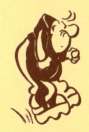

Beef Brisket

2-3 pounds lean beef brisket
3 1/2 cups beef broth
3 1/2 cups water
1 large onion, halved
3 carrots, sliced
2 celery stalks (including leaves), sliced
6 cloves garlic, minced
1 tablespoon parsley, chopped
Salt and pepper to taste

Place above ingredients in large pot and bring to boil. Simmer about 2 hours or until beef is tender. Skim the foam from the pot frequently. Remove all vegetables from pot with a slotted spoon, and discard.

6-8 small leeks, well trimmed
3 stalks celery, sliced diagonally
4 carrots, peeled and sliced
Salt and freshly ground pepper to taste

Add these vegetables (and any others you may like) to the beef and the broth. Season to taste. Cover and simmer until everything is very tender, at least 50 minutes. Slice beef diagonally to serve. Horseradish and stone ground mustard make nice condiments. Use the remaining broth as a gravy, or save to make hot sandwiches the next day.

6 servings (3 ounces)
per serving information
287 calories per portion
76.3 milligrams cholesterol
3.56 grams saturated fat
19.30 grams fat

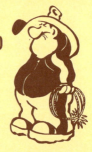

New England Boiled Dinner

3-5 pounds corned beef brisket
8-10 small onions
8 medium carrots
8 small new potatoes, skin on or off
1 medium green cabbage

Place brisket in large kettle, cover with cold water. Cover tightly. Simmer 4 to 5 hours or until tender. In a separate pot cook the onions, potatoes, and carrots. When they are just about done, add the cabbage and continue to simmer for 10 to 15 minutes.

10 servings
per serving information
281 calories
73 milligrams cholesterol
5.29 grams saturated fat
12.90 grams fat

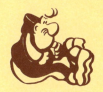

Mustard Barbequed Roast Beef

2 to 2-1/2 pound rib eye beef roast
1/2 to 1 cup Dijon mustard
2+ cups coarse Kosher salt

Insert a meat thermometer into the roast. Spread a thick coating of mustard over roast. Roll the roast in the salt, patting the salt into the mustard. Allow coals to reach "greyish" stage. Carefully place roast directly on the coals. Carefully turn the meat 1/4 turn every 10 minutes, placing it on fresh coals each time. Cook 25 minutes for rare, 30 minutes for medium rare, 35 minutes for medium well.

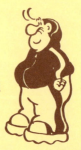

10 servings
per serving information
232 calories
68.87 milligrams cholesterol
4.936 grams saturated fat
13.70 grams fat

Beef Brisket Barbeque

5 pounds beef brisket, well trimmed
1 teaspoon salt
1/2 cup white onion, finely chopped
1/2 cup low-calorie catsup
1/4 cup red wine vinegar
1 tablespoon Worcestershire sauce
1 1/2 teaspoon liquid smoke
1 teaspoon freshly ground pepper

Preheat oven to 325°F.

Rub beef with salt. Place in ungreased 9x13" pan. Mix remaining ingredients and pour over beef. Cover and bake until tender, about 3 hours. Cut thin, diagonal slices. Spoon remaining juices over beef.

12 servings
per serving information
328 calories
123 milligrams cholesterol
6.09 grams saturated fat
17.00 grams fat

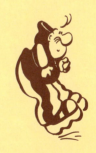

130   Main Courses

Our Favorite Beef Ribs

12 beef ribs
3 cups chili sauce
6 cloves garlic, minced
1/2 cup white onion, chopped
1/4 cup lemon juice
1/4 cup brown sugar
3 tablespoons Worcestershire sauce
1 teaspoon Dijon mustard
1 teaspoon Tabasco sauce
1 1/2 teaspoons freshly ground pepper

Preheat oven to 325°F.

Place the ribs in a tinfoil-lined shallow roasting pan. *Do not add salt or pepper!* Cover, cook in oven for 3 to 5 hours, until meat is very tender. Combine all other ingredients in saucepan and bring to boil. Reduce heat and simmer for 30 minutes. Remove ribs from oven and drain well.

There are 2 ways to serve:
1. Place ribs on individual plates and pass the sauce for dipping.
2. Arrange ribs in single layer in roasting pan. Brush each rib with sauce. Bake until sauce carmelizes, about 30 minutes.

6 servings
per serving information
424 calories
82.60 milligrams cholesterol
5.929 grams saturated fat
14.17 grams fat

Oriental Garlic Short Ribs

5 pounds beef short ribs, cut into 3/4-inch strips
4 cups water
1 1/2 cups lite soy sauce
1/2 cup sugar
15 cloves garlic, minced
1/2 cup green onions, thinly sliced
4 tablespoons sesame seeds
1 tablespoon sesame oil
2 tablespoons fresh ginger, minced
1 tablespoon honey
2 tablespoons Tabasco sauce

Place ribs in tinfoil-lined deep roaster. Combine remaining ingredients. Pour over ribs. Cover, refrigerate 24 hours. Turn ribs often. Broil or grill, turning only once.

10 servings
per serving information
422.5 calories
114.8 milligrams cholesterol
8.72 grams saturated fat
23.02 grams fat

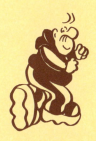

Low-Fat Beef Stroganoff

1 pound sirloin steak, well trimmed
      thinly sliced in strips
2 tablespoons flour
1/2 teaspoon freshly ground pepper
1 teaspoon olive oil
1 large white onion, chopped
2 cloves garlic, minced
12-15 mushrooms, thinly sliced
2 cups double-strength beef broth
3 tablespoons sherry or brandy
2 tablespoons tomato paste
1 teaspoon Dijon mustard
1/4 teaspoon oregano
1/4 teaspoon basil
1/4 teaspoon tarragon
1/2 cup plain low-fat yogurt

Sprinkle the flour and pepper over the steak. Toss to coat well. In a large, heavy skillet, heat oil. Saute onion, add garlic and mushrooms. Remove. Place meat in skillet and brown quickly. Return onions and mushrooms to skillet and add remaining ingredients, except yogurt. Cover, reduce heat, and simmer 20 minutes. Remove cover and allow to simmer 5 to 10 minutes longer. Add yogurt, mix well, and heat thoroughly. Serve over rice or hot cooked noodles. Garnish with parsley.

6 servings
per serving information
194.8 calories
51.79 milligrams cholesterol
3.085 grams saturated fat
8.119 grams fat

Beer and Beef Stew

4 medium white onions, sliced
2 tablespoons olive oil
2 pounds lean sirloin steak or tip,
    cut into 1-inch cubes
2 12-ounce cans beer
1 cup water
1 tablespoon corn syrup
1/2 teaspoon salt
1/2 teaspoon thyme
1/2 teaspoon marjoram
1 teaspoon freshly ground pepper
2 tablespoons cornstarch
1/4 cup cold water

Preheat oven to 350°F.

Saute onions in oil in a large skillet or Dutch oven. Remove onions. Add beef and cook until brown, about 10 minutes. Add onion, beer, 1 cup water, corn syrup, salt, herbs, and pepper. Heat to boiling. Mix cornstarch and 1/4 cup cold water and gradually stir into beef mixture. Bring to boil. Cover and bake for 2 hours. Uncover and bake about 45 minutes longer.

10 servings
per serving information
214.8 calories
55.7 milligrams cholesterol
3.4 grams saturated fat
13.70 grams fat

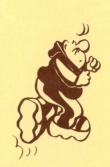

Burgundy Beef

2 tablespoons olive oil
2 white onions, sliced
1 pound fresh mushrooms, sliced
2 pounds round steak, lean, well trimmed,
      cut into 1-inch cubes
1/2 teaspoon garlic
1/2 teaspoon Italian seasoning
1/4 teaspoon thyme
1 teaspoon fresh ground pepper
1 1/2 tablespoons flour
3/4 cup beef broth
1 1/2 cups hearty red Burgundy

Heat oil in a heavy skillet. Brown meat. Add seasonings and herbs. Mix flour and broth, stir into skillet. Heat to boiling, stirring constantly. Boil and stir 1 minute. Add wine. Cover and simmer 2 to 2 1/2 hours or until meat is tender. Liquid should always cover meat. If necessary, add more wine and broth (1 part broth to 2 parts wine). Saute onions and mushrooms and add to beef. Cook for an additional 15 minutes. Garnish with chopped parsley.

6 servings
per serving information
328 calories
84.20 milligrams cholesterol
2.99 grams saturated fat
11.50 grams fat

Red Wine Sirloin Skillet

2 tablespoons margarine
1 cup green onions, chopped
1/4 cup shallots, chopped
1/2 teaspoon dried thyme
1 1/2 cups dry red wine
3-4 pounds boneless top sirloin steak, well
      trimmed, cut about 1 1/2-inches thick
2 tablespoons butter
4 tablespoons parsley
1 tablespoon lemon juice
1 tablespoon all-purpose flour

In a large heavy skillet, melt margarine over medium-high heat. Saute onions, shallots, and thyme about 2 to 3 minutes. Add wine and cook until reduced by 1/3. Remove sauce from skillet. Sear steak for 1 1/2 minutes on both sides. Turn heat to medium and let skillet cool slightly. Add sauce, remaining margarine, and parsley. Mix lemon juice and flour, and add to skillet. Cook for an additional 2 to 4 minutes per side.

Slice steak in diagonal strips 1/2 to 2 inches wide. Serve remaining sauce on the side.

6 servings
per serving information
160 calories
25 milligrams cholesterol
2.03 grams saturated fat
7.19 grams fat

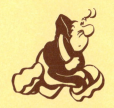

Fajitas

**1 pound top round steak, well trimmed,
     sliced 1/4-inch thick**
1/3 cup lime juice
3 cloves garlic, minced
1 teaspoon Mrs. Dash™ seasonings
1/2 teaspoon freshly ground pepper
1 tablespoon olive oil
1 large white onion, sliced
4 tortillas, warmed
1 cup lettuce, shredded
1 cup tomato, chopped
1/4 cup green onions, thinly sliced
1/4 cup cheddar cheese, grated
8 teaspoons sour cream

Combine lime juice, garlic, Mrs. Dash™ seasonings, and pepper. Place steak in glass bowl, add marinade, toss. Cover and refrigerate for 6 to 8 hours, stirring occasionally. Drain steak well. In a skillet, heat oil, saute onion. Add beef and brown. To serve, place an equal amount of meat, onion, lettuce, tomato, green onion, cheese, and sour cream on each warm tortilla.

4 servings
per serving information
398 calories per serving
87.63 milligrams cholesterol
7.357 grams saturated fat
19.77 grams fat

Marcos Mexican Steak Tartar

2 pounds very fresh, finely ground filet of beef
1/2 cup fresh chili pepper (serrano or jalepeño) finely chopped
3 cups white onion, finely chopped
3 cups ripe tomatoes, finely chopped (a green tomato, finely chopped is a nice addition)
1 cup cilantro, chopped
Freshly ground pepper
Worcestershire sauce
20 limes, halved
Parsley to garnish

Place 3 ounces of ground steak on each plate. Arrange the other ingredients around the filet. Add Worcestershire sauce, pepper, and lime juice to individual taste.

8 servings
per serving information
261 calories
95.3 milligrams cholesterol
4.5 grams saturated fat
10.80 grams fat

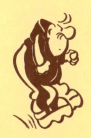

Simple Spaghetti Sauce

3 medium white onions, chopped
2 tablespoons margarine
2 green peppers, chopped
3 stalks celery, sliced diagonally
2 teaspoons fresh parsley, chopped
2 medium carrots, sliced
3 pounds ground beef, lean
Salt and freshly ground pepper to taste
1 32-ounce can tomato sauce with
     Italian seasoning
1 12-ounce can tomato paste with Italian seasonings
1-2 teaspoons Italian seasonings

Saute onions in margarine until light brown. Add other vegetables. Simmer 5 minutes. Remove from slillet. Brown meat quickly, season with salt and pepper. Add vegetables, tomato sauce, and tomato paste. Add water if sauce is too thick (beer can be substituted for the water). Simmer at least 1 hour. Serve over hot spaghetti noodles. Garnish with parsley and Romano cheese.

12 servings
per serving information
278 calories
75.94 milligrams cholesterol
4.368 grams saturated fat
11.60 grams fat

Thick Meat Sauce

1 large white onion, chopped
10 cloves garlic, minced
2 tablespoons olive oil
1 1/2 pounds ground beef, lean
1 6-ounce can tomato paste
2 14-ounce cans Italian stewed tomatoes
1 cup red wine
Freshly ground pepper
1 pound fresh mushrooms, thinly sliced
2 teaspoons oregano
2 teaspoons Italian seasoning
Parmesan cheese to garnish

In a large, heavy skillet heat oil over medium heat. Saute the onion until translucent, add garlic, and saute 1 minute. Remove onion and garlic, brown ground beef. Drain thoroughly. Return onion, garlic, and meat to skillet. Add other ingredients. Simmer 1 to 2 hours.

Serve over spaghetti noodles. Garnish with parsley and Parmesan cheese.

10 servings
per serving information
217 calories
43 milligrams cholesterol
2.8 grams saturated fat
8.97 grams fat

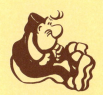

Porcupines

1 pound ground beef, lean
1/2 cup rice, uncooked
1/2 cup water
1/2 cup onion, chopped
1 teaspoon garlic salt
1/2 teaspoon celery salt
1/2 teaspoon pepper
1 16-ounce can tomato sauce
1 cup water
2 teaspoons Worcestershire sauce

Heat oven to 350°F.

Mix meat, rice, 1/2 cup water, onion, salts, and pepper. Form into tablespoon-sized balls. Place in ungreased baking dish. Stir together remaining ingredients, pour over meat balls. Cover and bake 45 minutes. Uncover and continue baking 15 minutes more.

6 servings
per serving information
278 calories
63.10 milligrams cholesterol
4.90 grams saturated fat
12.70 grams fat

Spanish Rice with Meat

1 pound well-trimmed lean beef, cubed
1 medium onion, finely chopped
1 teaspoon garlic, minced
3/4 teaspoon paprika
1/2 cup green peas, dried
1 red pepper, cut in strips
2 cups long grain white rice
1 large tomato, cut in medium-sized pieces
1 tablespoon olive oil
Salt and pepper to taste

Heat the oil in a large skillet and brown the onion and garlic. Season with salt and paprika. Stir. Add the beef and saute until well browned. Cover the meat with water and add the peas. Cover the pan and cook slowly until the meat is tender and the peas are cooked. Calculate the amount of water left in the pan and add sufficient water to cook the rice (approximately 4 cups liquid to 2 cups rice, or according to package proportions). Bring to boil and add the rice, strips of red pepper, and tomatoes. Cover the pan and cook slowly until the rice is done.

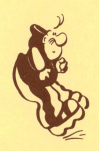

8 servings
per serving information
303 calories
37.97 milligrams cholesterol
2.37 grams saturated fat
7.12 grams fat

142   Main Courses

Texas Skillet Supper

1 pound ground sirloin, lean
1 cup white onion, chopped
2 10-ounce cans stewed tomatoes
1 4-ounce can chili peppers, chopped
1 16-ounce can pinto beans with jalapeño peppers,
      drained
4 cloves garlic, minced
2/3 cup long grain white rice
1 teaspoon chili powder
1/2 teaspoon red pepper flakes
1/2 cup Monterey Jack or cheddar cheese

In a heavy skillet, lightly brown beef, add onions, and cook until tender. Saute garlic. Drain fat. Stir in tomatoes, chilies, beans, rice, and spices. Add 1 cup water. Bring to a boil. Reduce heat, cover, simmer about 25 minutes or until rice is cooked. Garnish with cheese and parsley sprigs.

6 servings
per serving information
357 calories
45.20 milligrams cholesterol
4.35 grams saturated fat
14.30 grams fat

Curried Sweet Potato and Beef

2 teaspoons olive oil
1 cup white onion, coarsely chopped
4 cloves garlic, minced
1 pound lean, well-trimmed beef, cut in 1-inch cubes
2-4 teaspoons curry powder, depending on taste
1/4-1/2 teaspoon cayenne pepper
12 ounces sweet potatoes, peeled, cut into
    1/2-inch slices
2 teaspoons fresh ginger, chopped
2 ripe tomatoes, cut in wedges
1 14-ounce can beef broth
1 package frozen pea pods, thawed

In a large skillet saute the onion and garlic in oil. Brown the meat. Add the curry, cayenne, and potatoes. Stir lightly until all ingredients are coated with the curry powder. Add the ginger, tomatoes, and broth. Cover and simmer about 20 minutes. Add the pea pods, cover, and simmer until pea pods are heated through.

6 servings
per serving information
239 calories
46.60 milligrams cholesterol
2.86 grams saturated fat
8.13 grams fat

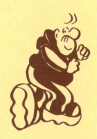

Stuffed Green Peppers

3 large firm green peppers
1/2 pound ground beef, lean, well trimmed
1/2 cup cracker crumbs
1/4 cup onion, chopped
1/2 teaspoon salt
1/2 teaspoon fresh ground pepper
1 8-ounce can of tomato sauce with Italian spices

Preheat oven to 350°F.

Cut thin slice from stem end of each pepper. Remove all seeds and membranes. Wash inside and outside. Mix remaining ingredients. Lightly stuff each pepper with 1/3 of the meat mixture. Place in baking dish. Cover. Bake 45 minutes. Uncover, bake 15 minutes longer.

3 servings
per serving information
264 calories
64.60 milligrams cholesterol
5.12 grams saturated fat
13.40 grams fat

Beef Stuffed Tomatoes

1 pound ground steak
1 small white onion, chopped
4 large tomatoes
1 medium zucchini, peeled, shredded, and drained
1/2 cup low-fat Mozzarella cheese, shredded
1/4 cup Parmesan cheese
1/4 cup Italian bread crumbs
4 cloves garlic, minced
Generous grinding of fresh pepper

Combine beef and onion, arrange in a ring in microwave-safe sieve or colander. Place sieve in microwave-safe bowl and microwave on high for 4 minutes, breaking up beef after 2 minutes. Stir beef after removing from oven. Scoop out each tomato. Combine the beef mixture with all the other ingredients. Put an equal portion in each tomato. Place tomatoes in a microwave-safe dish. Cook on high for 6 minutes, rotating after 3 minutes.

4 servings
per serving information
360 calories per serving
87 milligrams cholesterol
9.7 grams saturated fat
22.50 grams fat

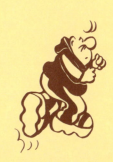

Shepherd's Pie

1 pound ground beef, lean
   or left-over roast beef, ground
2 white onions, chopped
4 cloves garlic, chopped
4 teaspoons Worcestershire sauce
1 teaspoon parsley, chopped
1 teaspoon basil
1 teaspoon freshly ground pepper
2 cups mashed potatoes

Preheat oven to 350°F.

In a heavy skillet, brown beef (this is not necessary if using left-over roast). Add onion and garlic. Cook until lightly browned. Add Worcestershire sauce, parsley, basil, and pepper. Simmer 5 minutes. Spray baking dish with non-stick vegetable spray. Place beef mixture in baking dish, cover with mashed potatoes. Sprinkle with paprika. Bake for 1 hour. Garnish with parsley.

6 servings
per serving information
212 calories
51.96 milligrams cholesterol
3.003 grams saturated fat
7.276 grams fat

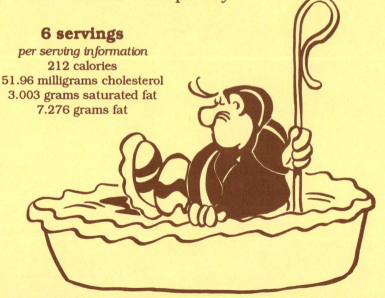

Hungarian Goulash

2 tablespoons olive oil
2 cups white onions, chopped
3 pounds top sirloin steak, boneless, well trimmed
Freshly ground pepper
1 tablespoon margarine
1 tablespoon olive oil
1/4 cup low-calorie catsup
3 tablespoons paprika
1/4 teaspoon garlic salt
4 cloves garlic, minced
1 can condensed beef broth
1/3 cup red wine
1 cup low-fat yogurt

In a large, heavy skillet or Dutch oven, heat oil and saute onions until translucent. Remove and set aside. Add margarine and freshly ground pepper. Add meat and brown quickly. Add the sauteed onions and the other ingredients except the yogurt. Blend well. Cover tightly and simmer 1 to 2 1/2 hours until meat is tender. Finally, blend the yogurt into the sauce and heat thoroughly. Garnish with parsley.

12 servings
per serving information
267 calories
77.3 milligrams cholesterol
4.9 grams saturated fat
26.50 grams fat

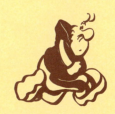

Sunday Morning Hash

1 pound ground sirloin steak, or left-over
     roast beef, ground
2 large white onions, chopped
2 cloves garlic, minced
16 mushrooms, quartered
4 large potatoes, peeled, boiled, and cubed
3 tablespoons Worcestershire sauce
1 can lite beer
Freshly ground pepper

In a heavy skillet, brown beef, remove, and drain well. Pour off excess fat, add onions, and saute. Add garlic, potatoes, Worcestershire sauce, and heat thoroughly. Return beef to pan, add beer to moisten. Cook about 5 minutes, continuing to add beer as needed. Garnish with parsley. (The cook can drink the remaining beer.)

Variations: Add diced green chilies and serve with salsa.

8 servings
per serving information
213.5 calories
37.87 milligrams cholesterol
2.126 grams saturated fat
5.37 grams fat

Entertaining with Beef

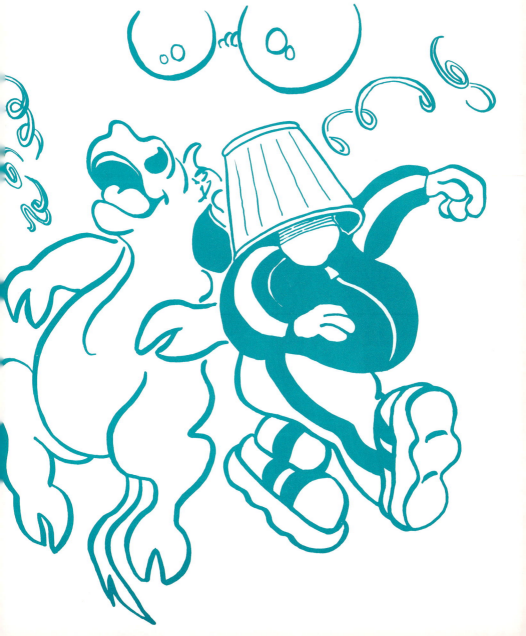

151

Menu 1   152
   Beef Artichoke Salad
   Horseradish Dressing
   Broiled Fruit Kabobs

Menu 2   154
   Beef Tenderloin Dianne
   Snow Pea Salad
   Fettuccini with Onion-
     Wine Sauce
   Lime Sherbet

Menu 3   156
   Steak au Poivre
   Italian Mushrooms
   Twice Baked Potatoes
   Green Salad with Garlic
     Yogurt Dressing
   Polka Dot Melons

Menu 4   158
   Filet Mignon with
     Lemon Garlic Accent
   Wild Rice Pilaf
   Sauteed Snow Peas
     and Cucumbers
   Sweet and Sour
     Broccoli
   Bananas Foster

Menu 5   160
   Southwestern Grilled
     Steak
   Mexican Potatoes
   Fresh Salsa
   Green Salad with
     Parsley Dressing
   Fresh Fruit Dessert

Menu 6   162
   Hawaiian Flank
     Steak
   Chinese Style
     Vegetables
   Fresh Fruit Dessert
     with Aloha Sauce

Menu 7   164
   Spaghetti Squash with Wine Meat Balls
   Green Salad with Dilly Buttermilk
     Dressing
   Poached Apples

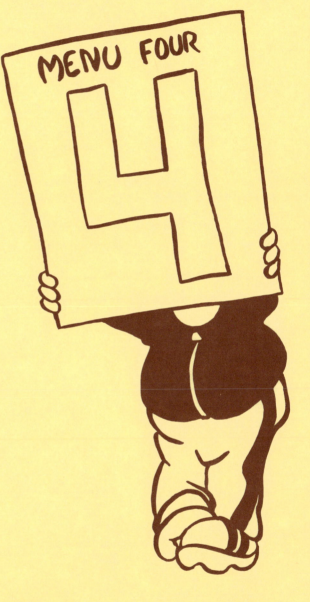

152   Menus for Four

Menu 1

per serving information
427.14 calories   81.19 milligrams cholesterol

Beef Artichoke Salad

**6 spinach leaves, washed, stems removed
3 ounces roast beef, well trimmed, finely sliced
1 small carrot, cut into sticks
4 artichoke hearts
4 small mushrooms, finely sliced**

Arrange the spinach leaves on a plate. Place the artichokes in the middle and alternate rolled beef and carrot sticks in spoke design. Arrange mushrooms around artichokes. Garnish with parsley.

1 serving   75.94 milligrams cholesterol
per serving information   4.230 grams saturated fat
277.7 calories   10.82 grams fat

Horseradish Dressing

**1 tablespoon light mayonnaise
1 tablespoon plain low-fat yogurt
1/4 teaspoon horseradish**

Combine all ingredients and chill well.

1 serving   5.25 milligrams cholesterol
per serving information   0.016 grams saturated fat
48.44 calories   4.026 grams fat

Broiled Fruit Kabobs

1/4 cup honey
1 1/2 teaspoons lemon juice
A variety of fresh or canned fruit cut into 3/4-inch cubes. Try pineapple, kiwis, kumquats, oranges, grapefruit, or pears.

Preheat oven to broil.

Blend honey and lemon juice.

Soak bamboo skewers for 1 hour. Arrange the fruit on long bamboo skewers, place on a well greased rack in the broiler pan. Brush the dressing on the fruit. Broil kabobs about 5 to 6 inches from broiler 1 to 2 minutes or until light brown. Turn, brush again with dressing, broil an additional 1 to 2 minutes.

1 serving (1 skewer)
per serving information
101 calories

0.0 milligrams cholesterol
.038 grams saturated fat
0.49 grams fat

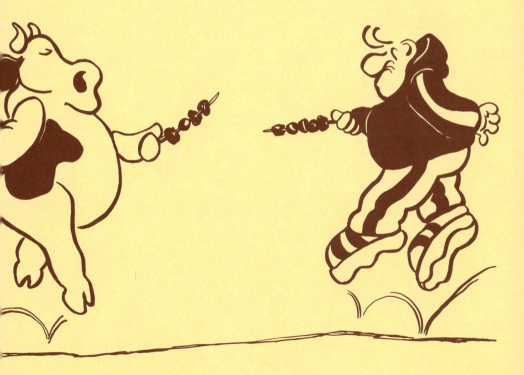

Menu 2

per serving information
705.9 calories   105.27 milligrams cholesterol

Beef Tenderloin Dianne

4 beef tenderloin steaks, 1 1/2-inch thick
1/4 teaspoon freshly ground pepper
1 tablespoon margarine
1 tablespoon olive oil
2 teaspoons lemon peel, grated
2 tablespoons fresh lemon juice
2 tablespoons Worcestershire Sauce
1/2 teaspoon garlic powder
1 teaspoon Dijon mustard

Pound steak to 1-inch thick. Sprinkle both sides with pepper. In a heavy skillet, over medium heat, melt margarine, add olive oil, and lemon peel. Add steaks and fry 6 to 8 minutes. Turn only once. Remove steaks, keeping them warm. Add remaining ingredients to skillet. Cook about 3 minutes, scraping skillet thoroughly. Pour over steaks. Garnish with parsley.

4 servings   84 milligrams, cholesterol
per serving information   4.131 grams saturated fat
243.9 calories   12.86 grams fat

Snow Pea Salad

1 pound snow peas, well trimmed
1 tablespoon olive oil
1 tablespoon sesame seeds, toasted
1 teaspoon sugar
1 1/2 tablespoons balsamic vinegar
1/2 - 3/4 teaspoon lite soy sauce

Cook the pea pods in a small amount of water until they are crisp tender, 1 to 2 minutes. Rinse in cold water and drain well. In a small skillet, heat the oil, add the seeds, then add the vinegar, sugar, and soy sauce. In a glass bowl combine the dressing and peas. Coat well. Serve chilled.

4 servings   0.0 milligrams cholesterol
per serving information   .524 grams saturated fat
93 calories   4.71 grams fat

Menus for Four   155

Fettuccini with Onion Wine Sauce

4 tablespoons margarine
5 large white onions, halved, thinly sliced in circles
2 carrots, peeled, thinly sliced
2 cloves garlic, minced
1/4 teaspoon salt
1/2 cup white wine (bourbon may be substituted)
1 1/2 cups chicken broth
1/2 teaspoon freshly ground pepper
8 ounces fettuccini
Parmesan cheese and parsley to garnish

In heavy skillet melt 3 tablespoons margarine over low heat. Add onions, carrots, and garlic. Cover and cook slowly, stirring often, about 1 hour. Add salt, wine, and broth. Continue cooking about 10 minutes. Toss pasta with remaining margarine. Cook fettuccini according to package directions. Toss pasta and onion sauce lightly, sprinkle with pepper, and garnish with cheese and parsley.

4 servings	17.9 milligrams cholesterol
per serving information	1.2 grams saturated fat
232 calories	7.21 grams fat

Lime Sherbet

2/3 cup boiling water
1 envelope low-calorie, sugar-free gelatin, lime flavor
1/2 cup sugar
1 1/2 cups buttermilk
1 1/2 teaspoon grated lemon peel
2 tablespoons fresh lemon juice

Pour boiling water over gelatin and sugar in glass bowl, stirring until both are dissolved. Mix in remaining ingredients. Chill in freezer until thickened. Beat until foamy. Pour into sherbet glasses. Freeze until firm.

4 servings	3.37 milligrams cholesterol
per serving information	.81 grams saturated fat
137 calories	.52 grams fat

156　Menus for Four

Menu 3

per serving information
656.15 calories　76.98 milligrams cholesterol

Steak au Poivre

1 pound sirloin steak, 2 inches thick, well trimmed
1 tablespoon olive oil
1/4 cup cracked pepper
3/4 cup dry red wine
1/2 cup brandy
1/4 cup double-strength beef broth
16 mushrooms, thinly sliced and sauteed

Press pepper into both sides of steak. Heat oil in heavy skillet. Add steaks and sear for 1 minute per side. Reduce heat and cook steaks 6 minutes per side for rare, 9 minutes per side for medium. Transfer steaks to warmed platter. Pour off any excess fat in skillet. Add wine and brandy, scraping all the sides of skillet. Add broth and continue cooking over high heat about 4 to 5 minutes. Slice steak, top with mushrooms, and pour sauce over all. Garnish with parsley.

4 servings	75.94 milligrams cholesterol
per serving information	4.603 grams saturated fat
283.9 calories	13.50 grams fat

Italian Stuffed Mushrooms

1 pound large fresh mushrooms
1 bunch fresh green onions
3 tablespoons fresh parsley, chopped
1 teaspoon Italian herbs
4 tablespoons margarine

Preheat oven to 425°F.

Clean mushrooms, removing stems. Clean the stems and chop finely. Mix the chopped stems with the other ingredients. Fill the mushroom caps with the mixture. Bake for about 15 minutes or until the top begins to brown.

24 mushrooms	0.0 milligrams cholesterol
per mushroom information	.178 grams saturated fat
13.75 calories per mushroom	1.04 grams fat

Twice Baked Potatoes

2 6-ounce baking potatoes, soaked, scrubbed
1/4 cup skim milk
2 tablespoons margarine
1 teaspoon parsley, chopped
1 teaspoon chives, chopped
1/2 teaspoon garlic powder
Freshly ground pepper

Bake potatoes until easily pierced by fork. Cut off thin lengthwise slice. Scoop out potatoes, leaving a 1/4-inch shell. Mash potatoes and mix in the remaining ingredients. Spoon mixture into shells. Return to oven and cook until top is slightly browned. Garnish with parsley.

2 servings	.5 milligrams cholesterol
per serving information	1.07 grams saturated fat
208 calories	5.96 grams fat

Green Salad with Garlic Yogurt Dressing

Combine at least two different lettuces and top with sliced green onions and dressing.

1 tablespoon olive oil
1 tablespoon lemon juice
1/2 cup plain low-fat yogurt
1/2 teaspoon paprika
4 cloves garlic, minced
Dash of hot pepper sauce

Blend all ingredients in blender. Chill well.

2/3 cup	.182 milligrams cholesterol
per tablespoon information	.189 grams saturated fat
19 calories	1.27 grams fat

Polka Dot Melons

Cut a ripe cantaloupe in half, scoop out seeds. Cut each half lengthwise into wedges. With ball cutter, cut balls from wedges, replace with balls cut from a watermelon.

2 servings	0.0 milligrams cholesterol
per serving information	0.0 grams saturated fat
66 calories	0.73 grams fat

158   Menus for Four

Menu 4

per serving information
636 calories   76 milligrams cholesterol

Filet Mignon with Lemon Garlic Accent

4 filets of beef, well trimmed
5 teaspoons parsley, finely chopped
4 cloves garlic, minced
1/2 teaspoon lemon rind
1 teaspoon lemon pepper
Dash of garlic salt (optional)

Combine parsley, garlic, lemon rind, lemon pepper, and salt. Place the steaks on waxed paper and press the mixture into both sides. Cover and refrigerate at least 1 hour. On grill, cook steaks 6 minutes per side for medium. Or, using a heavy skillet sprayed with non-stick vegetable spray, cook 5 minutes per side.

4 servings   76 milligrams cholesterol
per serving information   3.4 grams saturated fat
195 calories   6.66 grams fat

Wild Rice Pilaf

1 medium white onion, chopped
1 teaspoon margarine
1 cup wild rice
3 cups water
1/2 teaspoon fresh ground pepper
1/2 teaspoon thyme
1 tablespoon fresh parsley, chopped

Saute onion in a large skillet with a tight-fitting lid, using the margarine and 1 tablespoon water. Add wild rice, water, and other seasonings except the parsley. Cook according to package directions, usually 20 to 25 minutes. Drain off any excess liquid. Serve with parsley garnish.

4 servings   0.0 milligrams cholesterol
per serving information   .151 grams saturated fat
185 calories   0.83 grams fat

Sauteed Snow Peas and Cucumbers

2 cucumbers, peeled, sliced
1/2 pound snow peas, washed, trimmed
2 tablespoons margarine
Ground pepper and mint leaves to taste

Saute cucumber and snow peas quickly (about 2 minutes). Sprinkle with mint and pepper to taste.

4 servings
per serving information
68 calories

0.0 milligrams cholesterol
.57 grams saturated fat
3.16 grams fat

Sweet and Sour Broccoli

1 pound broccoli with stems, cleaned, separated into flowerlets
2 tablespoons white sugar
4 tablespoons white vinegar
1 teaspoon salt
1 teaspoon sesame oil (optional)

Combine sugar, vinegar, and salt in an air tight container. Add the broccoli, making sure that it is well coated. Cover and refrigerate 12 hours, stirring occasionally. Drain before serving. Pour the sesame oil over just before serving.

4 servings
per serving information
65 calories

0.0 milligrams cholesterol
.22 grams saturated fat
1.52 grams fat

Bananas Foster

2 firm bananas
1 1/2 tablespoons margarine
2 tablespoons brown sugar, firmly packed
2 tablespoons dark rum
1/4 teaspoon cinnamon
1/8 teaspoon nutmeg

Peel bananas and cut into 1/4-inch slices. Melt margarine in 2-quart casserole. Stir in sugar, rum, and spices. Stir gently until sugar is melted. Add bananas and heat through. Serve at once.

4 servings
per serving information
123 calories

0.0 milligrams cholesterol
.48 grams saturated fat
2.41 grams fat

Menu 5

per serving information
537 calories   100.02 milligrams cholesterol

Southwestern Grilled Steak

1 pound sirloin steak, well trimmed
1/4 cup vegetable oil
Juice of 3 limes
6 cloves garlic, minced
Freshly ground pepper

Combine marinade ingredients. Blend well. Marinate steak for 6 to 18 hours, turning often. Grill over very hot coals. Slice diagonally to serve. Serve with salsa. Garnish with lime wedges and parsley.

4 servings   75.90 milligrams cholesterol
per serving information   4.11 grams saturated fat
202 calories   10.07 grams fat

Mexican Potatoes

1 pound potatoes, peeled and quartered
1/4 cup plain low-fat yogurt
1/4 cup skim milk
1/3 teaspoon chili powder
1/2 teaspoon red pepper flakes
1/4 cup parsley, chopped
1/4 cup green onions, finely sliced
1 4-ounce can chopped chilies, drained

Boil potatoes until tender. Drain well. Mash 1/2 of the potatoes. Add the other ingredients to the mashed potatoes, return both the mashed mixture and the potato pieces to a saucepan. Place over low heat and cook until heated thoroughly. Garnish with parsley or a light sprinkling of grated cheddar cheese.

4 servings   1.12 milligrams cholesterol
per serving information   .19 grams saturated fat
118.0 calories   .38 grams fat

Fresh Salsa

1 8-ounce can V-8 juice
4 ripe tomatoes, chopped
1 bunch green onions, chopped
1 small red onion, chopped
2 jalepeño peppers with seeds removed, finely chopped
Salt and freshly ground pepper to taste

Mix the above ingredients in a small glass bowl and chill for several hours before serving.

4 servings   0.0 milligrams cholesterol
per serving information   .047 grams saturated fat
48 calories   0.33 grams fat

Green Salad with Parsley Dressing

Combine several types of lettuce, radishes, and green onions. Toss lightly with parsley dressing.

1/2 cup olive oil
1/4 cup fresh lemon juice (approximately 3 lemons)
1 clove garlic, minced
1 egg
1 cup fresh parsley, chopped
Tabasco sauce to taste

Place all ingredients in blender. Process until thick and smooth. Serve over green salad, pasta, or cold cooked vegetables.

12 servings   23 milligrams cholesterol
per serving information   1.42 grams saturated fat
89 calories   9.48 grams fat

Fresh Fruit Dessert

1 cup cantaloupe balls.

1 serving   0.0 milligrams cholesterol
per serving information   0.0 grams saturated fat
80 calories   0.0 grams fat

162   Menus for Four

Menu 6

per serving information
366 calories   69.6 milligrams cholesterol

Hawaiian Flank Steak

1 pound flank or sirloin steak, well trimmed
1/4 cup frozen orange juice concentrate
2 tablespoons water
1 tablespoon corn syrup
1 tablespoon lite soy sauce
1/4 cup green onions, chopped
4 cloves garlic, minced
1/4 teaspoon ground ginger
Low-calorie canned fruit (pineapple rings, mandarin oranges, mixed fruits)

Combine orange juice, water, corn syrup, soy sauce, garlic, and ginger. Place steak in a sealed plastic bag. Pour marinade over steak and refrigerate 12 to 15 hours. Turn occasionally. Remove steak from marinade and either broil 4 to 5 minutes per side or grill it 5 to 6 minutes per side for medium rare. Slice diagonally across the grain into thin slices. Garnish with fruit and parsley.

4 servings   69.6 milligrams cholesterol
per serving information   3.77 grams saturated fat
185 calories   9.23 grams fat

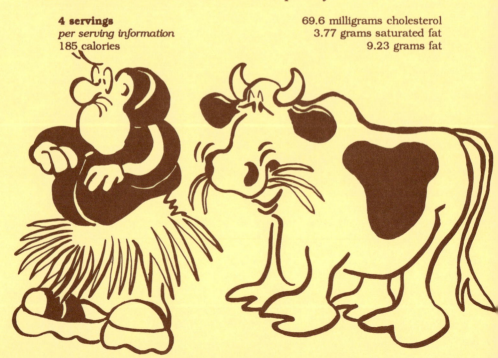

Chinese Style Vegetables

1 tablespoon water
3 cups cabbage, shredded
1 cup red onions, chopped
1 cup celery, chopped
1 medium green pepper, cut into circles
1 teaspoon salt
1 tablespoons lite soy sauce
Fresh ground pepper to taste

In skillet, mix water and vegetables. Cover, steam for 4 to 5 minutes or until vegetables are crisp yet tender. Season with salt, pepper, and soy sauce.

4 servings
per serving information
41 calories

0.0 milligrams cholesterol
.055 grams saturated fat
0.34 grams fat

Fresh Fruit Dessert

Arrange a selection of exotic fruits on a bed of lettuce and top with Aloha sauce.

1 cup fruit per person
per serving information
80 calories

0.0 milligrams cholesterol
0.0 grams saturated fat
0.0 grams fat

Aloha Sauce

2 tablespoons fresh lemon juice
1 tablespoon fresh lime juice
2 tablespoons fresh orange juice
1/3 cup water
1/3 cup sugar

This sauce is wonderful on melon salads, fruit, mixed green salads, and also on sausages, ham, and pork chops.

serving, 1 tablespoon
per serving information
20 calories per tablespoon

0.0 milligrams cholesterol
0.0 grams saturated fat
0.007 grams fat

164   Menus for Four

Menu 7

per serving information
424.7 calories   51.64 milligrams cholesterol

Spaghetti Squash with Wine Meatballs

2 pound spaghetti squash
3/4 pound lean ground beef
2 egg whites
1 tablespoon skim milk
1 tablespoon bread crumbs
2 tablespoons green onion, finely sliced
2 tablespoons parsley, chopped
1 tablespoon cornstarch
1 teaspoon beef granules
1 teaspoon catsup
1/4 teaspoon thyme
1/4 cup burgundy
Dash of garlic powder

Remove seeds from squash and cook until pulp can be pierced easily by a fork. Remove pulp and separate into strands. Keep warm.
Combine beef, egg whites, milk, bread crumbs, onion, and parsley. Shape into balls and bake for 20 minutes at 325°F. Drain well.
In a glass bowl, combine cornstarch and 2/3 cup water. Add other ingredients. Transfer to saucepan and cook over low heat until mixture thickens. Add meatballs, heat thoroughly. Serve over spaghetti squash, garnish with parsley and freshly ground pepper.

4 servings   49.4 milligrams cholesterol
per serving information   4.7 grams saturated fat
266.7 calories   12.1 grams fat

Menus for Four   165

Green Salad with Dilly Buttermilk Dressing

Arrange a selection of seasonal greens on individual plates. Garnish with thinly sliced kiwis and radishes. Top with dressing.

1 cup buttermilk
1 teaspoon white onions, minced
1 teaspoon chives, chopped
1 teaspoon parsley, chopped
1/4 teaspoon dried dill weed
1/2 teaspoon Dijon mustard
2-3 cloves garlic, minced

Blend all ingredients in blender. Chill well.

1 cup
per serving (per tablespoon) information
7 calories

.56 milligrams cholesterol
.084 grams saturated fat
0.15 grams fat

Poached Apples

1 cup apple juice
2 tablespoons raisins
1/4 teaspoon ground nutmeg
1/4 teaspoon cinnamon
2 teaspoons cornstarch
4 small green apples

Combine juice, raisins, and spices. Bring just to boil. Reduce heat. Core the apples and place in the saucepan also. Cover and simmer about 5 to 8 minutes. Remove apples to serving dishes. Combine cornstarch with a little cold water and stir into liquid. Cook and stir constantly until thickened. Cook at least 1 extra minute. Pour over apples.

4 servings
per serving information
130 calories per serving

0.0 milligrams cholesterol
.135 grams saturated fat
0.63 grams fat

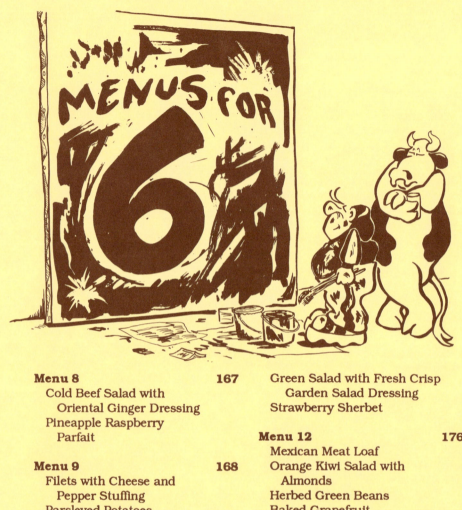

Menu 8 167	Green Salad with Fresh Crisp
Cold Beef Salad with	Garden Salad Dressing
Oriental Ginger Dressing	Strawberry Sherbet
Pineapple Raspberry	
Parfait	**Menu 12** 176
	Mexican Meat Loaf
Menu 9 168	Orange Kiwi Salad with
Filets with Cheese and	Almonds
Pepper Stuffing	Herbed Green Beans
Parsleyed Potatoes	Baked Grapefruit
Artichoke Salad	
Fresh Strawberries with	**Menu 13** 178
Grand Marnier	Beef Stuffed Baked Potatoes
	Italian Tomato and Zucchini
Menu 10 170	with Parmesan Cheese
Barbequed Filets with	Coleslaw
Tarragon Butter	Asparagus and Grape Salad
Tomato Aspic	Raspberry Sherbet
Summer Corn	
Green Salad with Cucumber	**Menu 14** 180
Salad Dressing	Meatballs and Noodles
Orange Souffle	Spinach and Broccoli
	Cucumber Salad with Green
Menu 11 174	Salad Dressing
Teriyaki Tips	Fresh Fruit Dessert with
Parsleyed Pasta	Raspberry Sauce

Menus for Six   167

Menu 8

per serving information
261 calories   50.63 milligrams cholesterol

Cold Beef Salad with Oriental Ginger Dressing

Sauce
3 cloves garlic, minced
2 teaspoons fresh ginger, minced
1 tablespoon sugar
1 tablespoon rice vinegar
1 tablespoon lite soy sauce
1 tablespoon vegetable oil

1 pound rare roast beef, well trimmed,
        thinly sliced, cut into julienne strips
1 green pepper, cut into strips
1 red pepper, cut into strips
1 cup green onions, thinly sliced
1 cup celery, thinly sliced
Shredded lettuce

Combine sauce ingredients in small jar and shake well. Arrange shredded lettuce on individual salad plates. Arrange vegetables and beef on top of lettuce. Spoon dressing over salad. Sprinkle with sesame seeds and parsley to garnish.

6 servings   50.63 milligrams cholesterol
per serving information   3.118 grams saturated fat
192 calories   9.303 grams fat

Pineapple Raspberry Parfaits

For each 1-cup serving, fill parfait glass with alternating layers of fresh raspberries and pineapple chunks. Pour low-calorie carbonated lemon-lime drink over fruit.

1-cup servings   0.0 milligrams cholesterol
per serving information   .037 grams saturated fat
69 calories   0.67 grams fat

168   Menus for Six

Menu 9

per serving information
592 calories   84 milligrams cholesterol

Filets with Cheese and Pepper Stuffing

**6 filets about 1-inch thick, well trimmed (make a pocket in each
       steak about 3 inches long, 1 1/2-inches deep)
1 cup onions, finely chopped
1 8-ounce can diced chili peppers, well drained
4 cloves garlic, minced
1 tablespoon olive oil
1/2 cup grated Monterey Jack or jalapeño cheese
Freshly ground pepper**

In a heavy skillet, heat oil and cook the onions until they are
translucent. Add garlic and chilies. Remove from heat. Add cheese
and a generous grinding of fresh pepper. Place 1/6 of the mixture in
each steak pocket and fasten with wooden toothpicks. Refrigerate if
prepared ahead. Grill steaks over medium coals about 6 minutes each
side for medium.

6 servings   84 milligrams cholesterol
per serving information   3.65 grams saturated fat
243 calories   10.90 grams fat

Parsleyed Potatoes

**2 pounds small new potatoes, either red or white
1/4 cup parsley, chopped
1 tablespoon lemon juice
Salt and freshly ground pepper**

Cover potatoes with cold water and bring to a boil over moderate heat.
Reduce heat and simmer 20 minutes or until fork tender. Drain. Stir
in other ingredients.

6 servings   0.0 milligrams cholesterol
per serving information   .039 grams saturated fat
134 calories   0.16 grams fat

Artichoke Salad

2 4-ounce cans of artichoke hearts, drained and halved
2 cups mushrooms, thinly sliced
1 1/2 cups snow peas, washed and trimmed
A bed of decorative lettuce (red salad bowl or bibb)

Dressing
1/4 cup red wine vinegar
1/4 cup virgin olive oil
2 teaspoons Dijon mustard
1 1/2 teaspoons garlic, minced
1 teaspoon dill weed
Fresh ground pepper to taste

In a glass bowl, combine vegetables.

Combine ingredients for dressing in a lidded jar and shake vigorously.
Pour dressing over vegetables. Toss well. Serve on a bed of lettuce.
Garnish with slivered almonds.

6 servings
per serving information
123 calories

0.0 milligrams cholesterol
1.02 grams saturated fat
7.14 grams fat

Fresh Strawberries with Grand Marnier

1 10-ounce package frozen raspberries, thawed
2 naval oranges, peeled
1 tablespoon Grand Marnier
2 pints fresh strawberries, washed and hulled

Puree raspberries and the liquid with them. Add 1/4 teaspoon of
orange zest from orange peel and the liqueur to the puree. Toss the
strawberries with the puree. Refrigerate. Arrange the orange slices on
a bed of fancy lettuce and top with the strawberries and puree.

6 servings
per serving information
92 calories

0.0 milligrams cholesterol
.019 grams saturated fat
0.31 grams fat

Menu 10

per serving information
476.40 calories   84.96 milligrams cholesterol

Barbeque Filets with Tarragon Butter

1/4 cup shallots or green onions, minced
2 tablespoons fresh parsley, chopped
5 teaspoons tarragon
Freshly ground pepper to taste
1/2 cup margarine
6 4-ounce filet steaks, well trimmed

Combine all ingredients except steak. Press into decorative butter molds or place in waxed paper and roll to form 1-inch round cylinder. Place in freezer until hard.

Grill or broil steaks. Slice margarine and place on top of steaks. Garnish with additional parsley.

6 servings   84 milligrams cholesterol
per serving information   4.965 grams saturated far
273.4 calories   16.90 grams fat

Tomato Aspic

1 1/4 cups boiling water
1 3-ounce package lemon or lime gelatin
1 8-ounce can tomato sauce or V-8™ juice
1 1/2 tablespoons vinegar
1/2 teaspoon garlic salt
1/2 teaspoon tabasco sauce
1/2 teaspoon onion juice
2 cups celery, diced
1/2 cup red onions, finely chopped

Pour boiling water over gelatin in a glass bowl. Stir until completely dissolved. Add tomato sauce, vinegar, and seasonings. Chill until it begins to thicken but is *not* set. Stir in celery and onion. Pour into 5 cup oiled mold. Chill until firm. Serve on a bed of lettuce with parsley garnish.

6 servings   0.0 milligrams cholesterol
per serving information   .006 grams saturated fat
25 calories   0.036 grams fat

Summer Corn

6 fresh cobs of corn, husked
1 tablespoon boiling water
3 teaspoons margarine, melted
1 teaspoon parsley, finely chopped
1/2 teaspoon paprika
1/4 teaspoon garlic salt
1/8 teaspoon ground red pepper

Cook corn. Mix remaining ingredients and brush mixture over corn. Keep corn hot in foil. These may also be made into bundles by dividing the mixture and wrapping each cob of corn separately and cooking on the grill.

6 servings
per serving information
92 calories per cob of corn

0.0 milligrams cholesterol
.323 grams saturated fat
1.96 grams fat

Green Salad with Cucumber Salad Dressing

Combine at least two different lettuces and top with sliced green onions and thinly sliced mushrooms.

1 cup low-fat yogurt
1/2 cup cucumber, seeded, peeled, and chopped, carefully drained
2 teaspoons chives, chopped
3/4 teaspoon dill weed
Dash of salt and freshly ground pepper to taste

Combine all ingredients and chill.

25 tablespoons
per serving (per tablespoon) information
6 calories

.16 milligrams cholesterol
.012 grams saturated fat
0.02 grams fat

Orange Souffle

3 egg whites
3 tablespoons sugar
1 teaspoon orange extract
2 tablespoons orange marmalade

Spray top and inside cover of 2 quart double boiler with non-stick vegetable spray. In a glass mixer bowl, beat the egg whites until foamy. Beat in the 3 tablespoons sugar, 1 tablespoon at a time. Continue beating until stiff. Beat in the orange extract. Fold in the orange marmalade. Pour into top of double boiler. Cover and cook over boiling water for 1 hour. *Do not remove cover.* Remove from heat, let stand until ready to serve, up to 30 minutes.

To serve, mound in individual serving glasses. Garnish with a tiny flower.

3 servings
per serving information
50 calories

0.0 milligrams cholesterol
0.0 grams saturated fat
0.0 grams fat

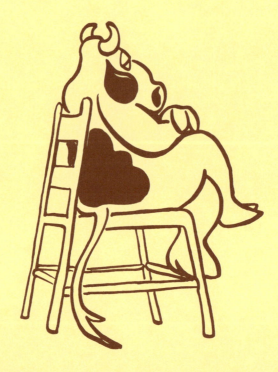

Remember...
Remain in Control!
*Develop an exercise program
which you enjoy.
If your exercise program is
burdensome,
you will soon abandon it.
Plan to exercise at a time
that is reasonable
and fits well with your
daily schedule,
thus helping to make
it easy to maintain.*

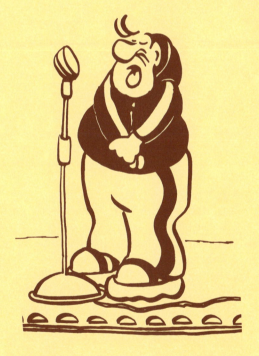

174   Menus for Six

Menu 11

per serving information
582.80 calories   93.63 milligrams cholesterol

Teriyaki Tips

**1 pound beef tip steak, well trimmed, 1/2-inch thick,
        cut into 6 serving-size pieces
1/4 cup sherry
4 tablespoons lite soy sauce
2 cloves garlic, minced
1 tablespoon olive oil
1/4 cup green onions, thinly sliced**

Combine sherry, soy sauce, and garlic. Marinate steak 1 to 2 hours.
In a heavy skillet, heat oil. Drain steaks, reserving marinade. Cook
steaks quickly, turning only once. Remove from heat. Add remaining
marinade to skillet and heat thoroughly. Pour over steaks. Garnish
with sliced green onions.

6 servings   50.63 milligrams cholesterol
per serving information   3.067 grams saturated fat
178.8 calories   8.983 grams fat

Parsleyed Pasta

**1 tablespoon olive oil
2 tablespoons shallots or green onions, chopped
1 pound fresh mushrooms, sliced
1 16-ounce can of Italian tomatoes, crushed
4 cups cooked pasta
1/2 cup low-fat ricotta cheese
1/4 cup Parmesan cheese, freshly grated
1/4 cup fresh parsley, chopped**

Heat oil in large skillet over moderate heat. Saute shallots. Add
mushrooms and cook 3 to 4 minutes. Add other ingredients and cook
until pasta is hot and the cheese is slightly melted. Garnish with
parsley before serving.

6 servings   43 milligrams cholesterol
per serving information   2.18 grams saturated fat
243 calories   6.91 grams fat

Green Salad with Fresh Crisp Garden Salad Dressing

Combine several types of lettuce, green peppers, and green onions. Toss lightly with dressing.

1/2 cup olive oil
1/4 cup tarragon vinegar
1/4 cup green onions, sliced
1/2 cup parsley, chopped
2 tablespoons green pepper, finely chopped
1 teaspoon garlic salt
1 teaspoon Dijon mustard
1/8 teaspoon tabasco sauce

Shake all ingredients in tightly covered jar. Refrigerate. Shake again at serving time.

serving, 1 tablespoon	0.0 milligrams cholesterol
ser serving information	.57 grams saturated fat
37 calories	4.03 grams fat

Strawberry Sherbet

2 teaspoons fresh lemon juice
2 large ripe bananas, cut into thin slices
2/3 cup unthawed frozen strawberries (unsweetened)
1/2 cup dietetic apple juice, chilled

Toss banana slices in lemon juice, arrange in single layer on waxed paper, cover, and freeze. Chop bananas and berries. Place in blender, add apple juice, and mix until smooth. May be refrozen in individual dishes or serve immediately. Garnish with mint leaves.

6 servings	0.0 milligrams cholesterol
per serving information	.075 grams saturated fat
50 calories	0.22 grams fat

Menu 12

per serving information
523.73 calories   55.92 milligrams cholesterol

Mexican Meat Loaf

1 pound lean ground beef
1/2 cup seasoned bread crumbs
1/2 cup skim milk
1 8-ounce can chopped green chilies
1 package taco seasoning
1 tomato, chopped
1/2 cup green onions, finely chopped
4 tablespoons salsa
1 4-ounce can diced green chilies
1/4 cup cheddar cheese, grated

Combine ground beef and bread crumbs. Mix well. Combine milk, chilies, and taco seasoning. Mix well. Blend both groups. Place mixture in loaf pan. Bake uncovered 1 hour at 350°F. Drain well, let stand 10 minutes, drain again. Combine remaining ingredients except cheese. To serve, slice meat loaf, top with salsa sauce. Garnish with cheese.

6 servings	55.92 milligrams cholesterol
per serving information	3.857 grams saturated fat
211.1 calories	9.060 grams fat

Orange Kiwi Salad with Almonds

3 naval oranges, peeled (save about 2 tablespoons peel)
3 kiwis, peeled, sliced
4 tablespoons Amaretto
2 tablespoons slivered almonds
1/4 cup golden raisins, soaked in 2 tablespoons orange liqueur

Cut the orange peel into julienne strips. Thinly slice the oranges. Arrange the fruit in alternating slices on a platter. Arrange peel lightly over the top. Drizzle fruit with Amaretto and top with almonds and raisins.

6 servings	00.00 milligrams cholesterol
per serving information	.138 grams saturated fat
108 calories	1.53 grams fat

Herbed Green Beans

1 pound fresh green beans
3 tablespoons margarine
2/3 cup white onions, chopped
1 clove garlic, minced
1/4 cup celery, chopped
1/4 cup parsley, chopped
1/4 teaspoon dried basil
1/4 teaspoon dried tarragon
Dash of salt
Freshly ground pepper to taste

Trim beans. Boil until crisp tender, about 10 minutes. Drain and keep warm. Melt margarine and lightly saute onion, garlic, and celery. Add parsley and herbs. Cover and simmer 10 minutes. Add beans and toss lightly.

6 servings
per serving information
60 calories

0.0 milligrams cholesterol
.557 grams saturated fat
3.13 grams fat

Baked Grapefruit

Cut 3 grapefruits in half. Remove seeds and loosen sections. Remove center. Sprinkle each half with 1/2 teaspoon granulated sugar and 1 teaspoon sherry. Chill 1 hour. Set oven control at broil.

Broil grapefruit 4 to 6 inches from heat 5 to 10 minutes until juice bubbles and edges of peel turn light brown. Serve hot. Garnish with a sprig of fresh mint.

6 servings
per serving information
51 calories

0.0 milligrams cholesterol
.017 grams saturated fat
0.12 grams fat

178   Menus for Six

Menu 13

per serving information
519 calories   39.39 milligrams cholesterol

Beef Stuffed Baked Potatoes

2 6-ounce baked potatoes
1/4 cup beef broth
1/4 cup onion, finely chopped
1 tablespoon parsley, chopped
1 tablespoon Worcestershire sauce
1/3 cup skim milk
Fresh ground pepper to taste
1 cup lean ground beef

Cut the potatoes in half and remove the pulp. Mash the pulp. Saute the parsley and onion in the beef broth. Add the ground beef and the Worcestershire sauce and cook until the beef is browned. Add the skim milk to the mashed potatoes. Combine the meat and potato mixtures, adding pepper to taste. Continue to cook until heated thoroughly. Reassemble potatoes and return to the oven for 5 minutes at 500°F.

2 servings   26.00 milligrams cholesterol
per serving information   1.49 grams saturated fat
244 calories   9.47 grams fat

Italian Tomato and Zucchini with Parmesan Cheese

1 tablespoon olive oil
2-3 cloves garlic, minced
3 cups zucchini, cut into half circles
1 cup ripe tomatoes, chopped, well drained
1 cup green onions, chopped, including tops
1/4 cup parsley, chopped
1/2 cup Parmesan cheese

Heat a large skillet, add oil, saute garlic for 20 to 30 seconds, add zucchini, saute for 2 minutes, add onions and saute until vegetables are crisp tender. Add tomatoes and parsley and heat thoroughly. Sprinkle with cheese. Toss lightly. Garnish with freshly ground pepper and parsley sprigs.

6 servings   6.5 milligrams cholesterol
per serving information   1.94 grams saturated fat
78 calories   4.92 grams fat

Coleslaw

3 cups cabbage, shredded
1 cup carrots, grated
1/3 cup red onion, grated
1/3 cup green pepper, finely chopped
1/3 cup plain nonfat yogurt
1/2 cup low-calorie mayonnaise
2 tablespoons cider vinegar
1 tablespoon Dijon mustard

Prepare vegetables. Mix other ingredients together. Whisk thoroughly. Add vegetables and toss.

6 servings
per serving information
85 calories per serving

6.89 milligrams cholesterol
.044 grams saturated fat
5.56 grams fat

Asparagus and Grape Salad

1 pound asparagus, trimmed
2 cups seedless green grapes, cut in half
1/2 cup red onion, chopped
2 tablespoons fresh tarragon, chopped
2 tablespoons vinegar
1 tablespoon olive oil

Blanch asparagus in large skillet of boiling water for 1 minute. Drain. Rinse in cold water, drain. Arrange asparagus and grapes on a serving platter. Mix the remaining ingredients and spoon over asparagus.

6 servings
per serving information
62 calories

0.0 milligrams cholesterol
.38 grams saturated fat
2.63 grams fat

Raspberry Sherbet

2 teaspoons fresh lemon juice
2 large ripe bananas, cut into thin slices
2/3 cup unthawed frozen raspberries (unsweetened)
1/2 cup dietetic apple juice, chilled

Toss banana slices in lemon juice, arrange in single layer on waxed paper, cover and freeze. Chop bananas and berries. Place in blender, add apple juice and mix until smooth. May be refrozen in individual dishes or serve immediately. Garnish with mint leaves.

6 servings
per serving information
50 calories

0.0 milligrams cholesterol
.075 grams saturated fat
0.22 grams fat

180   Menus for Six

Menu 14

per serving information
379.7 calories   52.79 milligrams cholesterol

Meatballs and Noodles

1 pound ground steak, lean
1 tablespoon cornstarch
2 tablespoons Worcestershire sauce
2 tablespoons beef broth
1 teaspoon dried Italian herbs
4 cloves garlic, minced
1 large white onion, chopped
12 mushrooms, thinly sliced
1 1/2 cups double-strength beef broth
1/4 cup sherry
1/4 teaspoon thyme
Freshly ground pepper to taste
1/4 cup water
2 tablespoons cornstarch
3 tablespoons fresh parsley, chopped

Combine meat, cornstarch, Worcestershire sauce, broth, herbs, and garlic. Blend well. Form into 1-inch meatballs. Bake at 350°F for 18 minutes or until evenly browned. Drain well. In a heavy skillet, saute onions, and mushrooms. Add meatballs, broth, sherry, and herbs. Combine water and cornstarch and add to skillet, stirring constantly until thickened. Add 1/2 the chopped parsley. Serve over hot noodles. Garnish with the remaining parsley and freshly ground pepper.

6 servings   50.63 milligrams cholesterol
per serving information   2.779 grams saturated fat
187.7 calories   6.958 grams fat

Spinach and Broccoli

1 10-ounce package frozen spinach
1 10-ounce package frozen broccoli, chopped
1 small onion, finely chopped
2/3 cup water
1 tablespoon lemon juice

In covered pan, heat vegetables to boiling. Reduce heat, cook 5 minutes. Drain, toss with lemon juice. Add ground pepper to taste.

6 servings   0.0 milligrams cholesterol
per serving information   .03 grams saturated fat
31 calories per serving   0.19 grams fat

Cucumber Salad with Green Salad Dressing

2 small cucumbers, peeled, thinly sliced

Arrange cucumbers on bed of crisp lettuce. Spoon dressing on top. Garnish with Pansy Flowers if available.

Dressing
1 cup parsley
1 1/2 cups low-fat cottage cheese
1 tablespoon lemon juice
1 tablespoon skim milk
1/2 teaspoon basil
1/2 teaspoon salt
1/2 teaspoon freshly ground pepper
6-8 drops Tabasco sauce

Place all ingredients in blender. Cover and blend on high speed for 2-3 minutes. Chill.

serving, 1 tablespoon	.364 milligrams cholesterol
per serving information	.053 grams saturated fat
7 calories	0.089 grams fat

Fresh Fruit Dessert

1 cup seasonal berries

1 serving	0.0 milligrams cholesterol
per serving information	0.0 grams saturated fat
80 calories	0.0 grams fat

Raspberry Sauce for Just About Everything

1 cup fresh or frozen raspberries, unsweetened
1/3 cup orange juice
1 1/2 tablespoons sugar
2 teaspoons cornstarch

Thaw berries if frozen. Combine all ingredients in saucepan. Cook, stirring constantly, until sauce is thickened and bubbling. Cook at least 1 minute extra. If you wish, you may strain sauce to remove seeds. Cover and chill until serving time.

1 serving, per tablespoon	0.0 milligrams cholesterol
per serving information	.002 grams saturated fat
8 calories	0.03 grams fat

Remember...
Remain in Control.
Develop a system of personal positive reinforcement.
Pep talks to yourself, notes on the refrigerator announcing how many pounds are gone. Use whatever motivates you and keeps your spirits up.

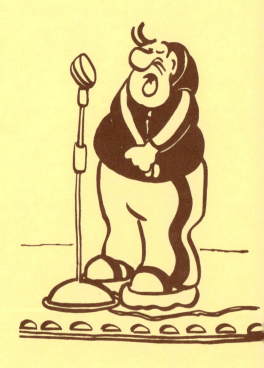

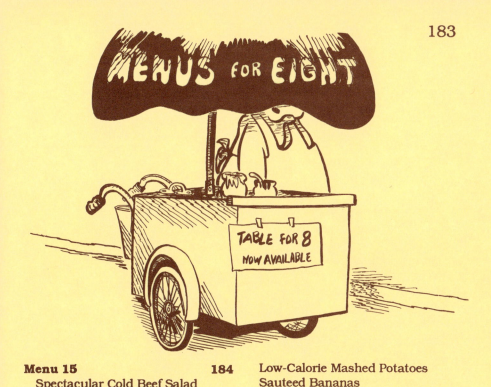

Menus for Eight

Menu 15 — 184
  Spectacular Cold Beef Salad
    with Caper Dressing
  Summer Peach Delight

Menu 16 — 186
  London Broil
  Overbaked Potatoes
  Caesar Salad
  Amazing Fake Chocolate
    Mousse

Menu 17 — 188
  Marinated Broiled Steak
  Wild Rice with Fresh Mushrooms
  Like Fresh Peas
  Cucumber Lemon Salad
  Fresh Fruit Dessert

Menu 18 — 190
  Italian Steaks
  Herb Broiled Tomatoes
  Green Onion Noodles
  Marinated Broccoli
  Strawberry Parfait

Menu 19 — 194
  Deluxe Pot Roast
  Green Salad with Creamy
    Spring Dressing
  Low-Calorie Mashed Potatoes
  Sauteed Bananas

Menu 20 — 196
  Meat Loaves
  Overnight Vegetable Salad
  Radish and Strawberry Salad
  Marinated Fresh Fruit

Menu 21 — 198
  Stuffed Zucchini
  Layered Vegetable Salad
    with Cottage Cheese Dressing
  Asparagus with Tart
    Vinaigrette Dressing
  Fresh Fruit Compote

Menu 22 — 202
  Albondigas Soup
  Cucumber and Orange Salad
  Mocha Angel Cake

Menu 23 — 204
  Mock Tenderloin
  Zucchini Mushrooms
  Stuffed Baked Potatoes
  Beefsteak Tomatoes in
    Spicy Dressing
  Raspberry Angel Food
    Delight

184   Menus for Eight

Menu 15

per serving information
426 calories   128 milligrams cholesterol

Spectacular Cold Beef Salad with Caper Dressing

1 1/2 pounds rare sirloin steak, well trimmed, sliced
        into thin strips
1/2 pound mushrooms, sliced
12-15 cherry tomatoes, cut in half
1 14-ounce can hearts of palm, sliced into rings
1 head of red lettuce
1 head of bibb lettuce
Fresh ground pepper
Selected Italian seasonings
1 red onion, sliced into rings, marinated separately

8 servings   57 milligrams cholesterol
per serving information   3.11 grams saturated fat
165 calories   7.74 grams fat

Caper Dressing

4 teaspoons capers
3 tablespoons fresh lemon juice
4 teaspoons Dijon mustard
1/2 cup red wine vinegar
1/2 cup virgin olive oil
1/4 teaspoon salt
Fresh ground pepper to taste
1 teaspoon sugar

Prepare Caper Dressing ahead and allow to refrigerate for 12 to 24
hours. Pour 1/3 of the dressing over the beef, refrigerate for 3 to 6
hours. Add other vegetables. Toss. Arrange on a bed of the mixed
lettuces. Garnish with thin slices of red onion, pepper, and seasonings. Serve additional dressing on the side.

                                          0.0 milligrams cholesterol
                                          1.92 grams saturated fat
per serving information   13.7 grams fat
122 calories

Summer Peach Delight

3 tablespoons white sugar
1 teaspoon white sugar
2 tablespoons cornstarch
1 cup low-fat milk
1 egg, separated
1 cup fresh peaches, peeled, sliced
2 tablespoons peach liqueur (Grand Marnier is nice too)
1 tablespoon fresh lemon juice
1/8 teaspoon either almond or orange flavoring

Combine 3 tablespoons sugar, cornstarch, and a dash of salt over low heat in a medium pan. Slowly stir in milk, beat in egg yolk. Beat until smooth, bring to boil, stirring constantly, boil 1 minute. In blender puree peaches, liqueur, lemon juice, and flavoring. Add to milk mixture. Place in glass bowl and cover tightly. Chill for at least 1 hour. Beat egg white until foamy, add 1 teaspoon sugar and beat until peaks form. Fold into peach mixture. Pour into 4 individual dishes. Cover and refrigerate. Garnish with mint leaves or little flowers.

4 servings
per serving information
139 calories

71 milligrams cholesterol
.824 grams saturated fat
2.08 grams fat

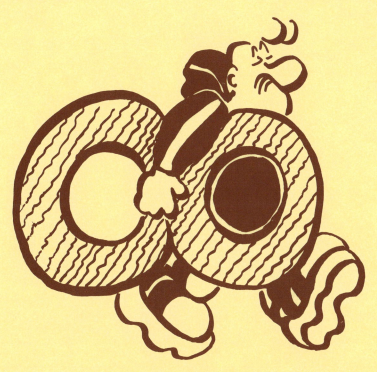

186   Menus for Eight

Menu 16

per serving information
665 calories   144.9 milligrams cholesterol

London Broil

1/4 teaspoon salt
2 tablespoons olive oil
1 teaspoon lemon juice
2-4 cloves garlic, minced
1/2 teaspoon freshly ground pepper
2 pounds high quality top sirloin or flank steak, well trimmed

Preheat oven to broil.

Stir all ingredients (except the meat) together. Brush on top side of the meat. Broil 2 to 3 inches from heat until brown (about 5 minutes). Turn meat and brush again with the oil mixture. Broil until rare, about another 5 to 6 minutes. To serve, cut into thin slices diagonally. Serve with Au Jus sauce and horseradish.

8 servings   75.9 milligrams cholesterol
per serving information   4.6 grams saturated fat
233 calories   16.80 grams fat

Overbaked Potatoes

2 6-ounce baking potatoes

Preheat oven to 450°F.

Wash potatoes well and pat dry. Pierce skin several times with a fork. Place potatoes on center rack of oven and bake 2 hours. Serve with freshly ground pepper.

2 servings   0.0 milligrams cholesterol
per serving information   .035 grams saturated fat
147 calories   0.20 grams fat

Caesar Salad

1 head Romaine lettuce, washed, torn into bite-sized pieces
3-4 cloves garlic, minced
1 teaspoon Dijon mustard
1-2 teaspoons Worcestershire sauce
1 teaspoon freshly ground pepper
1 lemon, juiced
2 egg whites
1 2-ounce can of anchovies, minced
1/2 cup green onions, chopped
1/2 cup olive oil
1/2 cup red wine vinegar
1/4 cup Parmesan cheese

Mix the above ingredients extremely well, except the lettuce and Parmesan cheese. Pour over Romaine lettuce that has been washed, patted dry, and chilled. Sprinkle with Parmesan cheese to taste. Both bacon bits and seasoned croutons can be added for a garnish.

8 servings
per serving information
164 calories

0.00 milligrams cholesterol
2.68 grams saturated fat
15.24 grams fat

Amazing Fake Chocolate Mousse

1/2 cup white sugar
1/3 cup unsweetened cocoa, sifted
1 teaspoon instant coffee
1/2 cup milk
3/4 cup milk
1 envelope unflavored gelatin
2 egg yolks, lightly beaten
1 teaspoon vanilla
4 egg whites

Combine 1/4 cup sugar, cocoa, coffee, and 1/2 cup milk in saucepan, add gelatin let stand 1 minute. Cook over medium heat until gelatin dissolves, stirring constantly. Combine 3/4 cup milk and egg yolks, add to gelatin mixture. Cook 5 minutes over medium heat, stirring constantly. Add vanilla, let cool. Beat egg whites until foamy, add remaining sugar, beat until stiff. Fold in cocoa mixture. Chill 3 to 4 hours.

8 servings
per serving information
121 calories

69 milligrams cholesterol
2.9 grams saturated fat
5.55 grams fat

188   Menus for Eight

Menu 17

per serving information
610 calories   77.15 milligrams cholesterol

Marinated Broiled Steak

2 pounds sirloin steak, well trimmed, about 1-inch thick
2 tablespoons olive oil
2 tablespoons lite soy sauce
1 tablespoon catsup
1 1/2 teaspoons dried basil leaves
1/2 teaspoon salt
1 teaspoon freshly ground pepper
1 teaspoon oregano
2 cloves garlic, minced

Place beef in large, flat container which is air tight. Mix remaining ingredients and pour over beef. Refrigerate for 4 to 6 hours, turning frequently. Place beef on rack in broiler pan. Broil 3 inches from heat, 7 to 8 minutes per side for medium. Slice diagonally about 1/3-inch thick.

8 servings   75.9 milligrams cholesterol
per serving information   4.6 grams saturated fat
237 calories   16.90 grams fat

Wild Rice with Fresh Mushrooms

2/3 cup wild rice
2 cups water
1/2 teaspoon garlic salt
1 cup mushrooms, cleaned and thinly sliced
2 teaspoons margarine

Rinse the rice well under cold water. Combine rice, water, and salt. Bring to boil, cover and simmer for 40 minutes. Add mushrooms, cover, and continue to simmer for 10 minutes. When all the liquid has been absorbed, add the margarine. It is possible to drain the rice if all the liquid is not absorbed, but the rice is tender.

4 servings   0.0 milligrams cholesterol
per serving information   .21 grams saturated fat
123 calories   1.19 grams fat

Menus for Eight   189

Like Fresh Peas

1 cup frozen peas
1 cup water
2 tablespoons white onion, finely chopped
1 tablespoon celery, finely chopped
1/8 teaspoon fresh mint (dried mint may be substituted)
Dash of salt and fresh finely ground pepper

Bring water to boil, add peas, onions, and celery. Cook about 3 to 4 minutes. Drain well. Add seasoning, mix well.

2 servings   0.0 milligrams cholesterol
per serving information   .045 grams saturated fat
66 calories   0.25 grams fat

Cucumber Lemon Salad

8 fresh mint leaves
8 fresh basil leaves
3 cucumbers, peeled and sliced thinly
8 ounces low-fat lemon yogurt
1/2 cup walnuts, chopped
1/2 cup golden raisins
1/2 cup green onion, chopped
1/4 cup green pepper, chopped

Chop mint and basil leaves. In a glass bowl combine all ingredients. Refrigerate several hours.

8 servings   1.25 milligrams cholesterol
per serving information   .436 grams saturated fat
104 calories   3.37 grams fat

Fresh Fruit Dessert

1 cup fresh berries

                                        0.0 milligrams cholesterol
per serving information   0.0 grams saturated fat
80 calories   0.0 grams fat

190   Menus for Eight

Menu 18

per serving information
512.80 calories   105.6 milligrams cholesterol

Italian Steaks

**8 filets, 4 ounces each, 1-inch thick
16 mushrooms, thinly sliced
4 cloves garlic, minced
6 ounces proscuitto, thinly sliced and then chopped
1/2 cup parsley, chopped
2 tablespoons fresh lemon juice
2 tablespoons olive oil
Freshly ground pepper**

Preheat oven to 500°F.

Spray baking dish with non-stick vegetable spray. Place mushrooms, garlic, proscuitto, and parsley in dish. Brush both sides of steak with oil. Place steaks in single layer on mushroom mixture. Bake for 8 minutes. Turn. Sprinkle with lemon juice and pepper. Return to oven 4 minutes for medium rare.

8 servings	87.78 milligrams cholesterol
per serving information	5.007 grams saturated fat
276.8 calories	14.77 grams fat

Herb Broiled Tomatoes

**4 large tomatoes, halved, with stem removed
1 teaspoon mixed Italian seasonings
1 teaspoon parsley, minced
Fresh ground pepper**

Preheat oven to 350°F.

Place tomato halves in baking dish and sprinkle with seasonings. Bake 20 minutes. Broil 2 to 3 minutes.

8 Servings	0.0 milligrams cholesterol
per serving information	.037 grams saturated fat
24 calories	0.26 grams fat

Green Onion Noodles

1/4 pound vermicelli noodles
1 tablespoon sesame oil
4 green onions, chopped very finely
1/4 teaspoon red pepper flakes

Cook noodles according to package directions. Drain. Add remaining ingredients. Toss. Serve at once.

4 servings
per serving information
102 calories

17.7 milligrams cholesterol
.476 grams saturated fat
4.12 grams fat

Marinated Broccoli

2 pounds fresh broccoli, well trimmed
1 whole head of garlic, peeled, minced
3 tablespoons lite olive oil
1/2 cup red wine vinegar (balsamic may also be used)
Salt and pepper to taste

Cook all ingredients in a large pot with a tight-fitting lid. Be sure all ingredients are just barely covered with water. Cook until broccoli is crisp and tender. Drain and refrigerate until well chilled.

8 servings
per serving information
76 calories

0.0 milligrams cholesterol
.781 grams saturated fat
5.45 grams fat

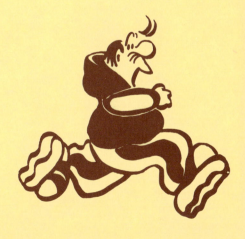

Strawberry Parfait

**20 fresh strawberries, washed, hulled, sliced
1/4 cup fresh strawberries, diced
1/4 ounce sugar-free strawberry gelatin
1/4 cup plain low-fat yogurt
1/2 cup whipped topping
1 teaspoon honey
1 teaspoon lemon rind**

Combine yogurt, whipped topping, diced strawberries, honey, and lemon rind. Combine 3/4 cup boiling water and ice cubes to make 1 1/4 cups and add to gelatin in a glass bowl. Stir until it starts to thicken. Remove any remaining ice cubes. This may now be assembled individually or in a medium-sized clear glass bowl. Place layer of strawberries and cover with about 1/3 of the gelatin mixture. Top this with all the yogurt mixture. Add a layer of the gelatin mixture and top with the remaining fruit. May also be made with raspberries or any combination of fruit except pineapple or banana (they brown if put on top).

8 servings
per serving information
34 calories

.125 milligrams cholesterol
1.04 grams saturated fat
1.36 grams fat

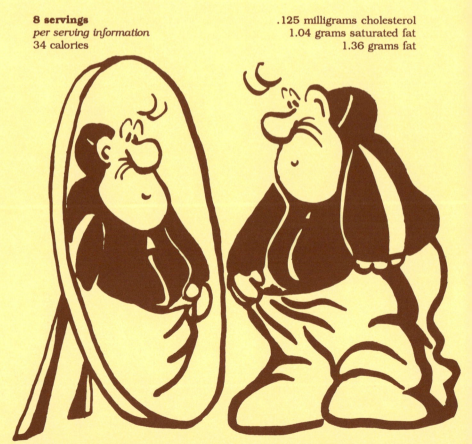

Remember...
Remain in Control!
Do not weigh every day. There is a three-day delay before what you eat affects your weight, and daily weight checks often prove more disappointing and frustrating than encouraging.

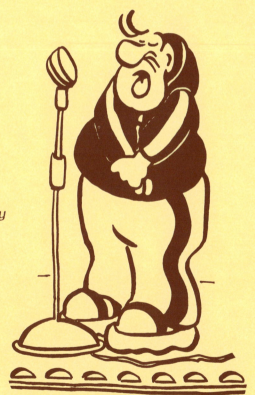

194   Menus for Eight

Menu 19

per serving information
616.6 calories   97.52 milligrams cholesterol

Deluxe Pot Roast

2 pound pot roast

Marinade
1/2 cup red wine
2 tablespoons olive oil
6 cloves garlic, minced
1/2 cup green pepper, chopped
1/2 cup white onion, chopped
1 teaspoon seasoned salt
1 teaspoon Mrs. Dash™ seasonings
1 teaspoon freshly ground pepper
2 tablespoons olive oil

1 6-ounce can tomato paste
1 teaspoon thyme
1 teaspoon oregano
1 teaspoon rosemary
6 ounces beer

Combine marinade ingredients. Pour over meat. Cover and refrigerate over night. Turn often. Drain well, reserving marinade. In a large Dutch oven, brown roast in 2 tablespoons olive oil. Add marinade, tomato paste, beer, and herbs. Simmer covered 3 hours. Serve with fresh steamed vegetables.

8 servings
per serving information
332.6 calories

90.15 milligrams cholesterol
6.290 grams saturated fat
20.04 grams fat

Green Salad with Creamy Spring Dressing

On a bed of crisp lettuce, arrange thinly sliced tomatoes, green peppers, radishes, and green onions. Pour dressing over salad.

1/2 cup low-calorie mayonnaise or salad dressing
2/3 cup buttermilk
2 cloves garlic, crushed
1 tablespoon chives or green onion, chopped
1 1/2 tablespoons parsley, chopped

Blend all ingredients and chill thoroughly.

8 servings
per serving information
50 calories

5.74 milligrams cholesterol
.112 grams saturated fat
4.19 grams fat

Low-Calorie Mashed Potatoes

1 1/2 pounds red potatoes with eyes and blemishes removed
1 teaspoon garlic salt
3/4 cup warm buttermilk
1/2 teaspoon baking soda
2 teaspoon margarine
1 clove garlic, minced
Freshly ground pepper to taste

Cover potatoes with cool water and add garlic salt. Boil until potatoes are tender, 45 to 50 minutes. Remove potatoes from water using a slotted spoon. Place in a large glass bowl and mash until fluffy, some lumps should remain. Mix the buttermilk and the baking soda together and mix into potatoes. If the potatoes are too dry, add 1 to 2 tablespoons of the cooking liquid. Stir in the garlic, the margarine, and the pepper. A little more salt may be added to taste.

8 servings
per serving information
116 calories

1.13 milligrams cholesterol
.309 grams saturated fat
1.02 grams fat

Sauteed Bananas

4 firm ripe bananas
1 1/2 teaspoons margarine
1/2 cup mango or peach puree
1/2 cup nonfat yogurt
Pinch of nutmeg
1 tablespoon nuts, finely chopped

Saute bananas in margarine 1 minute. Put slices of banana on individual plate with some mango or peach puree and some swirls of yogurt. Garnish with nutmeg and nuts.

50 calories
per serving information
118 calories

.5 milligrams cholesterol
.371 grams saturated fat
1.92 grams fat

196   Menus for Eight

Menu 20

per serving information
472.68 calories   75.24 milligrams cholesterol

Meat Loaves

12 ounces lean ground beef
2 tablespoons Italian bread crumbs
1/2 small onion, chopped
1 tablespoon nonfat milk
1 egg, lightly beaten
1 1/2 teaspoons prepared horseradish
2 cloves garlic, minced
1/4 teaspoon dill weed (optional)

Combine all ingredients, mixing thoroughly. Divide mixture into two equal portions and shape into loaves. Place loaves in microwave-safe baking dish. Cover with waxed paper and microwave on high 4 to 4 1/2 minutes, rotating dish after 2 minutes. Let stand 5 minutes before serving. Serve with Yogurt Dill Sauce.

4 servings   71.1 milligrams cholesterol
per serving information   5.5 grams saturated fat
248 calories   14.10 grams fat

Yogurt Dill Sauce

1/3 cup plain low-fat yogurt
1/4 cup cucumber, seeded, chopped
1 teaspoon onion, chopped
1/8 teaspoon dill weed
Dash of garlic salt

Combine all ingredients and chill well.

servings, 1 tablespoon   .125 milligrams cholesterol
per serving information   .009 grams saturated fat
5 calories   0.018 grams fat

Overnight Vegetable Salad

1 15-ounce can green beans
1 15-ounce can wax beans
1 2-ounce can chopped pimiento

1 red onion, chopped
1-2 stalks celery, sliced diagonally
1 medium green pepper, chopped
1 8-ounce bottle low-calorie ranch dressing

Drain canned vegetables, and place all vegetables in a glass bowl. Add dressing. Toss thoroughly. Cover, refrigerate at least 8 to 10 hours.

8 servings
per serving information
78.68 calories

3.544 milligrams cholesterol
0.776 grams saturated fat
3.909 grams fat

Radish and Strawberry Salad

1 cup radishes, thinly sliced
4 cups strawberries, hulled, sliced
1 cup green onions, including tops, chopped
1/4 cup red wine vinegar
2 tablespoons olive oil
3 cloves garlic, minced
1 head fancy lettuce

Combine oil, vinegar, and garlic, season with a little salt to taste. Lightly toss with the radishes, berries, and onions. Arrange on lettuce leaves on large platter. Drizzle any remaining dressing over the top. This recipe may also be used with cantaloupe rather than berries.

8 servings
per serving information
58 calories

00.0 milligrams cholesterol
.504 grams saturated fat
3.73 grams fat

Marinated Fresh Fruit

2 kiwi fruit, peeled, sliced
1 cup seedless green grapes
1 cup strawberries, halved
2 naval oranges, peeled, sliced
1 cup cantaloupe balls
3/4 cup orange juice
1/4 cup dry white wine
2 tablespoons fresh lemon or lime juice

Mix all ingredients in a glass bowl and chill for at least 3 hours.

8 servings
per serving information
63 calories

0.0 milligrams cholesterol
.018 grams saturated fat
0.33 grams fat

Menu 21

per serving information
541 calories   66.65 milligrams cholesterol

Stuffed Zucchini

3 pounds zucchini (either 2 large or 4 small)
1/2 pound ground beef, very lean
1 cup white onion, finely chopped
4-6 cloves garlic, minced
1/2 pound mushrooms, finely chopped
1/4 cup parsley, chopped
1/2 cup Italian bread crumbs
1/2 cup Parmesan cheese
1 egg, lightly beaten

Preheat oven to 375°F.

Trim the ends of the zucchini, slice them lengthwise, and remove the seeds. Parboil the zucchini halves for 6 to 8 minutes. Spray a heavy skillet with non-stick spray, heat, and lightly brown the beef. Add the onion and garlic, cook 3 minutes. Add the mushrooms and continue cooking for 5 minutes. Add the herbs and a generous grinding of fresh pepper. Remove from heat, stir in the egg and the bread crumbs. Divide the stuffing equally between the zucchini halves. Place in an appropriate size casserole that has been sprayed with non-stick vegetable spray. Sprinkle the cheese equally over the halves. A light sprinkling of red pepper flakes adds an extra tang.

8 servings   62.9 milligrams cholesterol
per serving information   3.28 grams saturated fat
145 calories   7.53 grams fat

Menus for Eight 199

Layered Vegetable Salad with Cottage Cheese Dressing

1 head crisp Boston lettuce
1 1-pound can beets, drained, sliced
1 cucumber, peeled, thinly sliced
1 large white onion, thinly sliced
2 large ripe tomatoes, thinly sliced
3-5 tablespoons chives, snipped

Dressing
1 pint low-fat cottage cheese
2 tablespoons light mayonnaise
1/2 teaspoon salt
1/2 teaspoon white pepper
1 tablespoons green onion, finely chopped

Combine all ingredients for dressing. Set aside. A clear, glass, straight-sided bowl is best. Place the chopped lettuce on the bottom of the bowl. Place the other ingredients in single layers in order given above. Top with the cottage cheese dressing and sprinkle with the chopped chives. Chill thoroughly.

8 servings
per serving information
88 calories

3.75 milligrams cholesterol
.412 grams saturated fat
1.86 grams fat

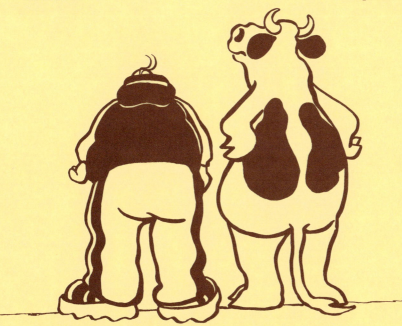

Asparagus with Tart Vinaigrette Dressing

48 fresh asparagus spears
1 head red leaf lettuce
8 strips pimiento

Trim asparagus into pieces 6 inches in length. Parboil in a large skillet about 5 to 7 minutes or until crisp tender. Drain and chill. Arrange asparagus in 8 separate bunches on a lettuce-covered tray and tie each bunch with the pimiento. Cover and return to refrigerator. Just before serving, pour Tart Vinaigrette Dressing over all.

Dressing
1/3 cup red wine vinegar
2/3 cup Italian olive oil
1 teaspoon salt
Fresh ground pepper to taste

Mix above ingredients in a jar and shake well. Refrigerate until serving time.

8 servings
per serving information
186 calories

0.0 milligrams cholesterol
2.6 grams saturated fat
18.2 grams fat

Fresh Fruit Compote

3 peaches, peeled, sliced
3 bananas, peeled, sliced
2 cups strawberries, sliced
2 cups blueberries
2 cups assorted melon balls
1 bottle (25 ounces) pink sparkling catawba grape juice

Assemble all fruit (except bananas) in a glass bowl. Cover tightly. Chill thoroughly. Just before serving, add bananas. Pour grape juice over.

8 to 10 servings
per serving information
122 calories per serving

0.0 milligrams cholesterol
.09 grams saturated fat
0.63 grams fat

Remember...
Remain in Control!
Establish short-term goals. They are the stepping stones to an ultimate goal. Make sure they are reasonable. Two pounds a week weight loss is an appropriate goal for most people.

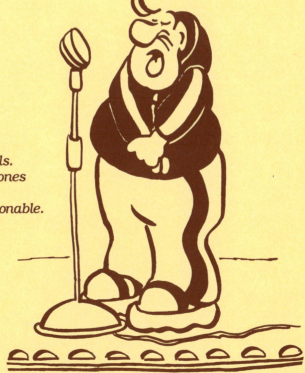

202   Menus for Eight

Menu 22

per serving information
358 calories   35.80 milligrams cholesterol

Albondigas Soup

2 tablespoons olive oil
1 large white onion, chopped
4-6 cloves garlic, chopped
2 10-ounce cans beef bouillon
1 7-ounce can diced green chilies
1 16-ounce can herbed tomato sauce
2 16-ounce cans stewed tomatoes
1 7-ounce can hot green chili salsa
2 teaspoons freshly ground pepper
1 teaspoon hot pepper sauce
1 teaspoon Mexican seasonings
1 1/2 pounds ground beef, made into 1-inch balls
1/2 cup red wine

Heat the oil in a large soup pot over medium heat. Add onion and garlic. Saute 3 to 4 minutes until translucent. Add bouillon, chilies, tomato sauce, stewed tomatoes, salsa, and seasonings. Heat to boil, then reduce heat and simmer for 1 hour. Add the meat balls and continue to simmer for 30 to 40 minutes. Add red wine 5 minutes before serving. Garnish with shredded cheddar cheese or parsley.

18 servings   33.80 milligrams cholesterol
per serving information   2.09 grams saturated fat
133.0 calories   6.42 grams fat

Cucumber and Orange Salad

1 cucumber, peeled, thinly sliced
1 15-ounce can dietetic mandarin orange sections, drained
1/4 cup low-calorie creamy cucumber dressing
Parsley to garnish

Toss all ingredients together, chill well, and garnish with parsley and freshly ground pepper. Serve on bed of lettuce.

4 servings
per serving information
83 calories

2.0 milligrams cholesterol
.425 grams saturated fat
2.21 grams fat

Mocha Angel Cake

Prepare an angel food cake mix following the directions on the package, except stir 1 tablespoon instant coffee into the dry mix before adding the egg whites. Top each slice with cut-up peaches and a sprinkle of nutmeg.

18 servings
per serving information
142 calories

0.0 milligrams cholesterol
.004 grams saturated fat
0.16 grams fat

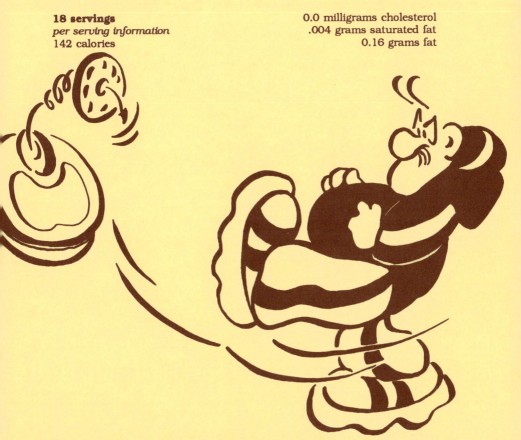

204   Menus for Eight

Menu 23

per serving information
738 calories   77.48 milligrams cholesterol

Mock Tenderloin

Trim 3 to 4 pounds lean eye of round roast

Preheat oven to 425°F.

Place meat thermometer so that it registers the thickest part. Place meat on rack in broiler pan. Cook meat for 50 to 55 minutes for rare (140°F on thermometer), 60 to 65 for medium (160°F). Remove from oven and let stand 10 minutes before serving. To serve, cut into thin slices.

12 servings   69.7 milligrams cholesterol
per serving information   3.1 grams saturated fat
173 calories   7.98 grams fat

Zucchini Mushrooms

20 large fresh mushrooms
3/4 cup zucchini, shredded
2 tablespoons green onions, sliced
1/3 cup fresh Parmesan cheese, grated

Heat oven to 375°F.

Clean the mushrooms, removing stems. Chop the stems. In a small skillet, combine chopped stems, zucchini, and onion plus 1 tablespoon water. Cook over medium heat until vegetables are tender. Drain. Stir in cheese. Divide the mixture evenly between the mushroom caps. Place in ungreased baking dish and bake for 10 minutes or until stuffing is browned and the mushrooms are tender.

serving, 1 mushroom   1.3 milligrams cholesterol
per mushroom information   .321 grams saturated fat
10 calories   0.53 grams fat

Stuffed Baked Potatoes

2 6-ounce potatoes, baked
1 medium onion, finely chopped
1/4 cup chicken stock (sodium free)
1/2 cup low-fat cottage cheese
2-3 tablespoons chives, chopped
Fresh ground pepper

Preheat oven to 350°F.

Cut the potatoes in half and remove the pulp. Mash the pulp. Saute the onion in the chicken broth. Add the mashed potato, cottage cheese, and pepper to the onion chicken stock mixture. Reassemble the potato halves and top with chopped chives. Return to oven for about 5 minutes.

2 servings
per serving information
204 calories

2.58 milligrams cholesterol
.45 grams saturated fat
0.98 grams fat

Beefsteak Tomatoes in Spicy Dressing

4 firm beefsteak tomatoes, sliced 1/4 to 1/2-inch thick
1 cup olive oil
1/2 cup red wine vinegar
2 teaspoons basil
2 teaspoons oregano
1 teaspoon salt
1 teaspoon freshly ground pepper
1/2 teaspoon Dijon mustard

Arrange tomato slices in large, flat dish. In a tightly covered jar, shake other ingredients. Pour over tomatoes. Cover. Chill for at least 4 to 5 hours. To serve, arrange tomatoes on bed of lettuce. Pour dressing over salad. Garnish with parsley.

10 servings
per serving information
152 calories

0.0 milligrams cholesterol
2.316 grams saturated fat
16.38 grams fat

Raspberry Angel Food Delight

3 cups fresh or frozen raspberries
2 tablespoons fresh lemon juice
3 tablespoons sugar
1 envelope unflavored gelatin
3/4 cup water
1 angel food cake loaf
1 1-1/4 ounce envelope low-calorie whipped dessert topping

Be sure to reserve a few berries for garnish. Crush remaining berries and add lemon juice. In a saucepan combine water, sugar, and gelatin. Heat and stir until gelatin and sugar are both dissolved. Allow to cool. Stir in raspberries. Chill slightly until partially set. Trim the cake loaf so that no brown remains and slice into 1/4-inch slices. Prepare topping mix according to package directions and add to raspberry mixture. Continue to chill until mixture mounds easily. Line a loaf pan with waxed paper. Arrange slices of cake around sides of pan. Add half the raspberry mixture. Top with cake slices. Add remaining half of mixture. Top with remaining cake slices. Chill thoroughly. Invert to serve. Garnish with remaining berries.

12 servings
per serving information
169 calories

0.0 milligrams cholesterol
.006 grams saturated fat
0.29 grams fat

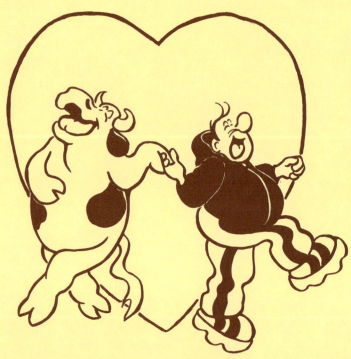

Party Menus 207

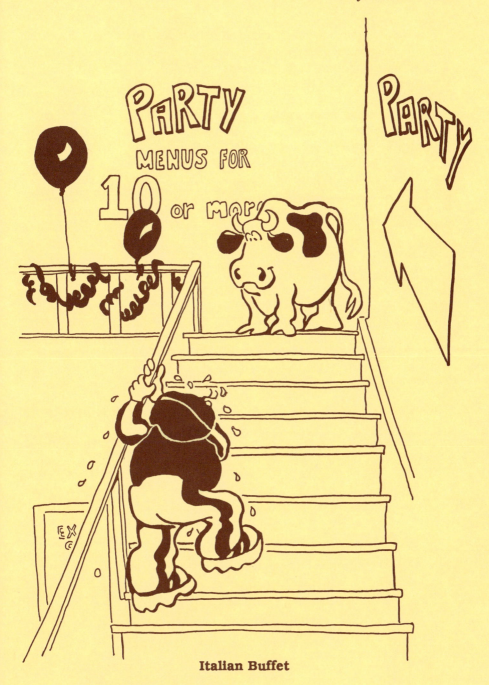

Italian Buffet

Low-Calorie Lasagne	209
Favorite Gazpacho	210
Cheese Dip with Vegetables	210
Melon Prosciutto Tidbits	211

Green Salad with Vinaigrette Dressing 211
Fresh Fruit Platter 211

Back Yard Picnic

Secret Marinated Chuck Roast 213
Fresh Onion Relish 214
"Let's Go Camping" Potato Salad 215
Three Bean Marinated Salad 215
Fresh Fruit Dessert 216
Oatmeal Squares 216

Barbeque

North Carolina Barbeque for a Crowd 217
Chili Dip 218
Vegetable Kabobs 218
Tequila Beans 219
Green Salad with Creamy Spring Dressing 219
Sweet Cereal Puffs 220

Beef Buffet

No-Fail Rib Roast 221
Horseradish Dip 221
Asparagus Wrapped in Proscuitto 222
Whole Roasted Onions 222
Spinach Cheese Casserole 223
Green Salad with Vinaigrette Dressing 223
Fresh Fruit Platter 224
Meringue Cookies 224

Cocktail Party

Simple Kabobs 225
Cheesy Fruit Dip 225
Chinese Beef Kabobs 226
Smoked Salmon Canapes 226
Oriental Meat Balls 227
Deviled Shrimp 227
Stuffed Mushrooms Caps 228
Crab Dip 228
Vegetable Dip 229
Fruit Nibblers 229

Italian Buffet

Low-Calorie Lasagne

8 lasagne noodles
3 9-inch zucchini, peeled and sliced lengthwise, 1/4-inch thick
1 1/2 pounds ground beef, lean
3 cloves garlic, minced
1 large white onion, chopped
1 28-ounce can Italian tomatoes with basil
1 16-ounce can Italian tomato sauce
Italian seasonings
1 teaspoon basil
2 teaspoons oregano
Fresh ground pepper to taste
1/2 cup red wine
Tabasco sauce to taste
16 ounces low-fat cottage cheese
8 ounces Parmesan cheese
2 tablespoons flour
8 ounces low-fat Mozzarella cheese
8 ounces Romano cheese

Preheat oven to 350°F.

Boil noodles according to package directions. Drain well. In a large skillet, brown meat. Remove and drain well. Remove excess fat from skillet, saute onions and garlic until translucent. Return meat to skillet. Add tomatoes and tomato sauce. Bring to boil, then reduce heat. Season to taste with Italian seasonings, basil, oregano, salt, freshly ground pepper, red wine, and Tabasco sauce. Simmer at least 1/2 hour. Spray 9x13" pan with non-stick vegetable spray. Combine Parmesan cheese, cottage cheese, and flour, and mix thoroughly. Place a layer of zucchini, followed by the cottage cheese mixture, then the meat sauce, and Mozzarella cheese. Repeat once. Add noodles on top, cover with meat sauce, and top with Romano cheese. Bake uncovered for 1 to 1 1/2 hours. Top should be lightly browned. Let stand 10 to 15 minutes before serving.

12 servings
per serving information
337 calories

66 milligrams cholesterol
8 grams saturated fat
15 grams fat

Favorite Gazpacho

1 16-ounce can Italian tomatoes, chopped
2 large ripe tomatoes, chopped
1 green pepper, chopped
1 cucumber, peeled and chopped
5 stalks celery, chopped
1 white onion, chopped
2 cloves garlic, minced
6 tablespoons red wine vinegar
4 tablespoons olive oil
20 ounces V-8 juice
Tabasco sauce to taste
Fresh ground pepper to taste

Mix all ingredients and allow to chill overnight.

12 servings   0.0 milligrams cholesterol
per serving information   .67 grams saturated fat
75 calories   4.69 grams fat

Cheese Dip

3 tablespoons sour cream
1 1/2 teaspoons Worcestershire sauce
1 clove garlic, minced
8 ounces low-fat sharp cheddar cheese, coursely grated
1/4 cup light beer, room temperature
Red pepper to taste
Broccoli, celery, cucumber or other vegetables to dip with

In top of double boiler, over boiling water, combine sour cream, Worcestershire sauce, and garlic. Add cheese slowly, stirring with wooden spoon. Stir in beer and pepper; heat until cheese is melted. Remove from water and let stand at room temperature while mixture thickens. Serve with cleaned, trimmed vegetables.

8 servings   32 milligrams cholesterol
per serving information   6.67 grams saturated fat
29 calories   10.50 grams fat

Melon Prosciutto Tidbits

1 honeydew melon
1/2 pound prosciutto

Cut melon in half, removing seeds. Cut each half into wedges and then slice the wedges into bite-size pieces. Cut the proscuitto into 1-inch strips. Wrap around melon chunks, securing with decorative toothpicks.

16 servings
per serving information
26 calories

7.4 milligrams cholesterol
.25 grams saturated fat
0.79 grams fat

Green Salad with Vinaigrette Dressing

Combine a selection of fresh salad greens. Toss lightly with vinaigrette dressing.

1/2 cup red wine vinegar
2/3 cup Italian olive oil
1 teaspoon salt
Freshly ground pepper

Combine in covered jar and shake thoroughly.

serving, 1 tablespoon
per serving information
84 calories

0.0 milligrams cholesterol
1.35 grams saturated fat
9.50 grams fat

Fresh Fruit Platter

Arrange a selection of fresh seasonal fruit on a bed of lettuce.

1-cup serving
80 calories

212   Party Menus

Party Menus   213

Back Yard Picnic

Secret Marinated Chuck Roast

4-5 pound chuck roast, at least 2 inches thick

Marinade
1 medium white onion, chopped
1 1/2 tablespoons olive oil
5 cloves garlic, minced
1/4 cup parsley, chopped
1 1/2 cups beef broth
3 tablespoons red wine vinegar
1/2 cup lite soy sauce
1 tablespoon brown sugar
1 teaspoon ginger
1 teaspoon allspice
1 teaspoon rosemary

Saute onion in oil, stir in remaining ingredients and bring to boil. Remove from heat and cool. Trim the roast and place in a deep casserole. Pour marinade over meat and marinate at least 12 to 15 hours, turning occasionally. Barbecue the roast over medium heat for 30 to 45 minutes.

10 to 12 servings   92.90 milligrams cholesterol
per serving information   4.38 grams saturated fat
264 calories   12.40 grams fat

Fresh Onion Relish

4 large white onions, cut in half and thinly sliced in circles
1/4 cup tarragon vinegar
2 tablespoons brown sugar
1 teaspoon freshly ground pepper
2 tablespoons fresh parsley, chopped
1 teaspoon fresh thyme, chopped

Spray a large heavy skillet with non-stick vegetable spray. Add onions and simmer about 1 1/2 hours, stirring frequently. Add remaining ingredients, continue stirring until thickened. May be served warm or at room temperature. Delicious with plain steak or roast beef.

serving, 1 tablespoon   0.0 milligrams cholesterol
per serving information   .013 grams saturated fat
15 calories   0.07 grams fat

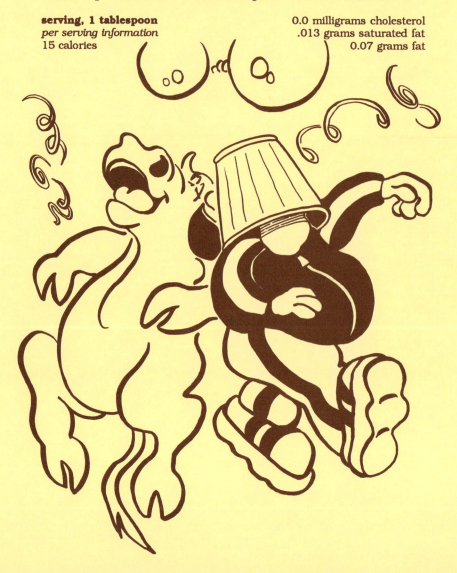

"Let's Go Camping" Potato Salad

2 pounds red potatoes, scrubbed and trimmed
1/2 cup green onions, including tops, finely chopped
1/2 cup light mayonnaise
1 tablespoon sugar
1 tablespoon tarragon vinegar
1 tablespoon Dijon mustard
1/2 teaspoon garlic salt
Generous grinding of fresh pepper
1/4 teaspoon celery seeds

Boil potatoes until tender. It is not necessary to peel them. Drain well and allow to cool. Combine all other ingredients in a large glass bowl. Add potatoes and toss well. Cover and refrigerate. Garnish with parsley and pimiento.

12 servings
per serving information
97.7 calories per serving

3.33 milligrams cholesterol
0.02 grams saturated fat
2.75 grams fat

Three Bean Marinated Salad

1 15-ounce can green beans
1 15-ounce can yellow beans
1 15-ounce can kidney beans
1/2 cup green peppers, chopped
1 medium red onion, thinly sliced in circles
1 tablespoon sugar
1/3 cup olive oil
2/3 cup red wine vinegar

Combine the sugar, oil, and vinegar, mixing well until the sugar is dissolved. Pour over the beans and vegetables. Chill overnight. Garnish with parsley to serve.

18 servings
per serving information
72 calories

0.0 milligrams cholesterol
.581 grams saturated fat
4.15 grams fat

Fresh Fruit Dessert

On a bed of lettuce, arrange a tray of seasonal fruits, including melon balls, sliced kiwis, green and red grapes, sliced oranges, and pineapple spears.

serving, 1 cup
per serving information
80 calories

0.0 milligrams cholesterol
0.0 grams saturated fat
0.0 grams fat

Oatmeal Squares

2/3 cup sugar
1/3 cup water
3 tablespoons vegetable oil
1/2 teaspoon vanilla
2 egg whites, beaten lightly
1/2 cup flour
1/3 cup quick-cooking oats, uncooked
1/4 cup cocoa, unsweetened
3/4 teaspoon baking powder
1/8 teaspoon salt

Preheat oven to 350°F.

Combine sugar, water, oil, and vanilla. Stir well. Add egg whites. Stir well. Combine flour, oats, cocoa, baking powder, and salt. Stir well. Add to sugar mixture. Stir well. Pour into 8x8" baking pan that has been sprayed with non-stick vegetable spray. Bake for 25 minutes or until wooden toothpick comes out clean.

15 servings
per serving information
79 calories

0.0 milligrams cholesterol
.374 grams saturated fat
2.87 grams fat

Barbeque

North Carolina Beef Barbeque for a Crowd
(Best made at least one day ahead)

10 pounds boneless beef brisket
1 cup liquid smoke
4 cups white onion, chopped
10 cloves garlic, minced
24 ounces tomato paste
5 cups light beer
1 28-ounce can Italian tomatoes
1 cup packed brown sugar
2/3 cup red wine vinegar
1/2 cup Worcestershire sauce
4 tablespoons chili powder
2 tablespoons molasses
1/2 teaspoon cloves
Freshly ground pepper

Preheat oven to 325°F.

Place racks in roasting pan. Put liquid smoke in bottom of pan beneath rack. Arrange meat on rack, do not allow meat to touch liquid. Cover. Bake until very tender, at least 4 1/2 hours, turning once. Refrigerate meat on rack in pan overnight.

Reserve all pan liquids, but only 1/4 cup of fat from surface. Place the 1/4 cup fat in large Dutch oven, add onion and garlic. Saute about 8 minutes. Add tomato paste. Measure reserved pan liquids, add enough beer to make 5 1/2 cups total. Add to onion mixture. Add all remaining ingredients except meat and additional beer. Cover. Simmer 1 hour, stirring often. Pull meat into 1-inch pieces. Add to sauce.

Cover. Simmer 1 hour. If sauce is too thick, add more beer. If sauce is too thin, remove cover and boil slightly. Serve on fresh buns. Garnish with parsley.

30 servings
per serving information
352.5 calories per serving

91.83 milligrams cholesterol
6.631 grams saturated fat
15.97 grams fat

Chili Dip

1 1/2 cups low-fat riccota cheese
1 tablespoon chili powder
1/2 to 1 teaspoon red pepper flakes
1/4 cup plain low-fat yogurt
1 tablespoon green onion, finely chopped
1 tablespoon parsley, finely chopped
1 4-ounce can chopped green chilies, drained

Combine all ingredients. Blend until smooth. Chill thoroughly. Serve with fresh vegetables.

yield, 2 cups, serving 1 tablespoon
per serving information
17 calories

3.5 milligrams cholesterol
.57 grams saturated fat
.92 grams fat

Vegetable Kabobs

1/2 pound beef salami
1 cantaloupe
1 6-ounce jar pickled mushrooms

Cube salami into 1/2-inch bite-sized pieces. Cut the melon in half, removing seeds. Using a melon baller, scoop the melon into balls. Alternate the salami, melon, and mushrooms on small bamboo skewers. Cover and refrigerate until chilled thoroughly.

1 kabob per serving
per serving information
31 calories

4.6 milligrams cholesterol
.641 grams saturated fat
1.63 grams fat

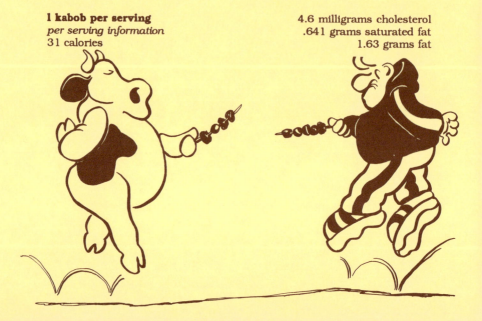

Tequila Beans

1 6-ounce can Italian tomato paste
1 15-ounce can dark kidney beans, drained
2 15-ounce jars of brick roasted pork and beans
2 15-ounce cans Italian stewed tomatoes
4 tablespoons brown sugar
3 tablespoons Dijon mustard
2 large white onions, chopped, sauteed
2 cups beef sausage, sliced diagonally
2 7-ounce cans diced chili peppers
1 1/2 cups tequila
2 teaspoons garlic, minced
Pepper to taste
1 to 2 teaspoons Cajun spices

Place all ingredients in large Dutch oven and simmer 6 to 8 hours, stirring often.

15 servings
per serving information
282.7 calories per serving

39 milligrams cholesterol
4.360 grams saturated fat
12.80 grams fat

Green Salad with Creamy Spring Dressing

On a bed of crisp lettuce, arrange thinly sliced tomatoes, green peppers, radishes, and green onions. Pour creamy spring dressing over salad.

1/2 cup low-calorie mayonnaise or salad dressing
2/3 cup buttermilk
2 cloves garlic, crushed
1 tablespoon chives or green onion, chopped
1 1/2 tablespoons parsley, chopped

Blend all ingredients and chill thoroughly.

8 servings
per serving information
50 calories

5.74 milligrams cholesterol
.112 grams saturated fat
4.19 grams fat

Sweet Cereal Puffs

3 egg whites
2/3 cup sugar
4 cups Total™ or Wheaties™ cereal

Preheat oven to 325°F.

In a large mixer bowl, beat egg whites until foamy. Beat in sugar, 1 tablespoon at a time. Continue beating until very stiff and glossy. Fold in cereal. Drop mixture by teaspoonfuls 2 inches apart onto a pan sprayed with non-stick vegetable spray. Bake 14 to 16 minutes.

4 dozen cookies *per serving information, one cookie* 20 calories	0.00 milligrams cholesterol .006 grams saturated fat 0.04 grams fat

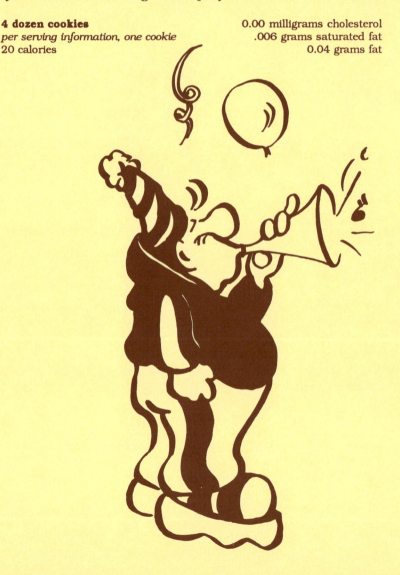

Beef Buffet

No-Fail Rib Roast

1 rib roast, any size, at room temperature

Preheat oven to 450°F.

Insert meat thermometer. Rub the roast with seasonings of your choice. Place in open roasting pan, rib side down. Roast at 450°F for 1 hour. Turn off oven. Do not open oven door. About 40 minutes before dinner, turn on oven again to 375°F. The meat will be well browned and rare inside. For better done meat or at high altitudes, add more time to the reheating. Check meat thermometer for correct degree of doneness.

3-ounce serving
per serving information
203.5 calories

68.87 milligrams cholesterol
4.936 grams saturated fat
11.72 grams fat

Horseradish Dip

1 cup low-fat cottage cheese
4 tablespoons Romano cheese
2 tablespoons chives, chopped
1 tablespoon parsley, chopped
3 tablespoons prepared horseradish
2 teaspoons fresh lemon juice
2 cloves garlic, minced
Dash of red pepper sauce

Combine all ingredients, stirring well. Cover and chill. Serve with fresh vegetables.

yield, 1 cup
per serving information
16 calories per tablespoon

2.64 milligrams cholesterol.
.057 grams saturated fat
0.68 grams fat

222   Party Menus

Asparagus Wrapped in Prosciutto

24 to 36 fresh asparagus stalks, well trimmed, steamed
8 thin slices proscuitto
1/2 cup Parmesan cheese
1/3 cup low-calorie margarine, melted
Freshly ground pepper

Preheat oven to 350°F.

Wrap 4 to 6 stalks asparagus in each slice of proscuitto. Secure with decorative toothpicks. Place them in a shallow baking dish that has been sprayed with non-stick vegetable spray. Sprinkle with cheese, drizzle margarine over the top. Bake 10 minutes. Allow to cool slightly before serving. Cut each bundle into 3 to 4 pieces, adding additional toothpicks if necessary.

6 servings   14.1 milligrams cholesterol
per serving information   2.83 grams saturated fat
139 calories   8.77 grams fat

Serve Fresh, Whole Wheat Rolls with Buffet

Whole Roasted Onions

24 small white onions (1 inch in diameter), peeled
2 tablespoons margarine
1 tablespoon parsley, finely chopped
2 tablespoons chives, finely chopped
1/4 teaspoon garlic salt
2 cloves garlic, minced

Preheat oven to 375°F.

Place onions in single layer in casserole that has been sprayed with butter flavored non-stick vegetable spray. Cover and bake in 375° oven for 45 minutes or until onions are tender. Melt margarine in heavy skillet over low heat. Add garlic and saute 30 seconds, add other ingredients, including onions, and heat thoroughly.

6 servings   0.0 milligrams cholesterol
per serving information   .353 grams saturated fat
32 calories per serving   2.02 grams fat

Spinach Cheese Casserole

2 cups low-fat cottage cheese
3 egg whites
1/3 cup flour
1 1/2 teaspoons Italian seasoning
4 cloves garlic, minced
Generous grinding of fresh pepper
6 cups fresh spinach, torn into bite-sized pieces
1 cup low-fat Mozzarella cheese, grated
1 8-ounce can water chestnuts, drained and sliced
1 large ripe tomato, thinly sliced

Preheat oven to 350°F.

Blend cottage cheese and egg whites until smooth. Combine flour, Italian seasoning, garlic, and pepper. Add cottage cheese mixture and combine well. Add spinach, 1/2 cheese and the water chestnuts. Pour mixture into an 8x8" casserole that has been sprayed with non-stick vegetable spray. Cover and bake at 350°F about 40 minutes or until a knife inserted comes out clean. Arrange the tomato slices over the casserole and sprinkle with the remaining cheese. Bake 5 minutes more or until the cheese is bubbly.

10 servings   10.60 milligrams cholesterol
per serving information   1.85 grams saturated fat
128 calories   3.10 grams fat

Green Salad with Vinaigrette Dressing

Combine a selection of fresh salad greens. Toss lightly with vinaigrette dressing.

1/2 cup red wine vinegar
2/3 cup Italian olive oil
1 teaspoon salt
Freshly ground pepper

Combine in covered jar and shake thoroughly.

serving, 1 tablespoon   0.0 milligrams cholesterol
per serving information   1.35 grams saturated fat
84 calories   9.50 grams fat

Fresh Fruit Platter

Arrange a selection of fresh seasonal fruit on a bed of lettuce.

Spoon low-fat pina colada yogurt over top. Garnish with fresh flowers.

per 1-cup serving of fruit
80 calories

Meringue Cookies

**3 egg whites
1 cup sugar
1/4 teaspoon salt
1 teaspoon vanilla**

Preheat oven to 300°F.

Blend egg whites, sugar, salt, and vanilla in top of a double boiler. Place over boiling water, beat with rotary beater, scraping bottom and sides of pan frequently until mixture forms stiff peaks. Drop mixture by teaspoonfuls onto baking sheet that has been sprayed with non-stick vegetable spray. (Two baking sheets will be required.) Bake only one at a time. Bake 12 to 15 minutes or until light golden brown. Remove immediately from baking sheet to cooling rack.

3 1/2 dozen cookies　　　　　　　0.0 milligrams per cookie
per serving information, 1 cookie　　0.00 grams saturated fat
18 calories　　　　　　　　　　　　0.00 grams fat

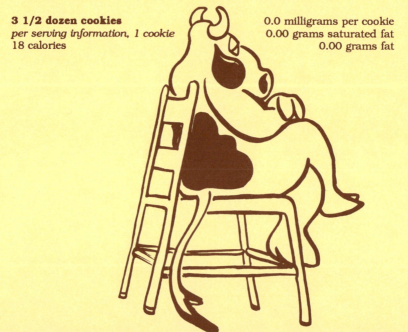

Cocktail Party

Simple Kabobs

1 pound sirloin steak cut into 1–inch cubes
1/2 cup calorie reduced Italian salad dressing
3 tablespoons lite soy sauce
4 cloves garlic, minced
1 teaspoon onion powder
8 mushrooms
8 cherry tomatoes
1 green pepper, cut into squares
1 small zucchini, cut into rounds

Place steak cubes in glass bowl. Combine next four ingredients. Pour over meat. Cover and refrigerate. Marinate at least 6 to 8 hours. Soak bamboo skewers for at least one hour. To assemble kabobs, alternate meat and vegetables on bamboo skewers. Broil or grill kabobs (about 5 minutes per side), brushing with marinade frequently.

4 servings (2 skewers per serving)   77.94 milligrams cholesterol
per serving information   4.571 grams saturated fat
270.7 calories   13.44 grams fat

Cheesy Fruit Dip

2 cups dry, low-fat cottage cheese
2/3 cup skim milk
2 teaspoons chives, chopped
2 teaspoons fresh lemon juice
1/2 teaspoons salt
A selection of fresh fruits cut into bite-size pieces

Mix all ingredients (except fruits) in blender until smooth. Cover and chill 4 to 5 hours. Arrange fruits on a bed of lettuce with dip on the side.

serving, 1/3 cup   2.9 milligrams cholesterol
per serving information   .389 grams saturated fat
49 calories   0.61 grams fat

Chinese Beef Kabobs

1/2 cup hoisin* sauce
2 tablespoons white wine
1 tablespoon vegetable oil
6 cloves garlic, minced
2 teaspoons fresh ginger, minced
1 teaspoon Chinese five spice powder
1 1/2 pounds sirloin steak, well trimmed, thinly sliced

Soak bamboo skewers for at least 1 hour. Combine all ingredients except meat. Blend well. Thread meat onto skewers. Place in shallow pan and brush with sauce. Grill about 3 minutes per side, basting constantly. Sprinkle with sesame seeds to serve.

24 skewers
serving information per 1-ounce skewer
57.30 calories

18.98 milligrams cholesterol
1.110 grams saturated fat
3.085 grams fat

*Available in the oriental spice section of your supermarket.

Smoked Salmon Canapes

1 6-ounce package smoked salmon
1 fresh cucumber, peeled
1 4-ounce package lite cream cheese
1 red onion, sliced paper thin
Capers for flavor and garnish

Slice the cucumber into 1/4-inch rounds. Lightly cover each round with cream cheese. Divide the salmon equally, placing on top of the cheese. Place several small pieces of onion atop the salmon and nestle capers between to hold them in place. A few drops of fresh lime juice is a nice addition.

20 servings
per serving information
35 calories

7.715 milligrams cholesterol
.989 grams saturated fat
1.99 grams fat

Oriental Meat Balls

2 pounds ground steak
1 teaspoon garlic powder
1 teaspoon freshly ground pepper
2 ounces water chestnuts, chopped
3 green onions, finely chopped
3 tablespoons terriyaki sauce

Mix all ingredients, form into 1-inch balls, and saute in skillet until browned. Drain on paper towel. May be served plain or with low-calorie Russian dressing.

12 servings
*per serving information*1
119 calories

45.9 milligrams cholesterol
.23 grams saturated fat
3.50 grams fat

Deviled Shrimp

2 pounds large raw shrimp
1 lemon, thinly sliced
1 red onion, thinly sliced
1 cup pitted black olives, well drained
2 tablespoons pimiento, chopped
1/4 cup olive oil
3 cloves garlic, crushed
1 tablespoon Dijon mustard
4 tablespoons lemon juice
1 tablespoon red wine vinegar
Dash of cayenne
4 tablespoons parsley, chopped

Shell and clean shrimp. Cook shrimp in boiling salted water for 3 minutes only. Drain at once, rinse in cold water, drain well. In a glass bowl, combine lemon slices, onion, black olives, and pimeiento. Toss well. Combine the other ingredients in a separate bowl and then add to the lemon mixture. Arrange the shrimp on a tray and pour dressing over them. Cover and chill up to 3 hours. Serve with fancy toothpicks.

30 servings
per serving information
50.24 calories per serving

59.2 milligrams cholesterol
.349 grams saturated fat
2.224 grams fat

Stuffed Mushroom Caps

1 pound large fresh mushrooms
1 tablespoon fresh garlic, minced
4 tablespoons fresh parsley, chopped
1/2 teaspoon Italian herbs
1/4 pound margarine, softened

Clean mushrooms, removing stems. Mix other ingredients. Fill each mushroom cap with mixture. Broil until filling is bubbling.

24 servings
per serving information
23 calories per serving

0.0 milligrams cholesterol
.349 grams saturated fat
2.01 grams fat

Crab Dip

1 teaspoon sugar
1/4 teaspoon white pepper
1/3 cup lite cream cheese
1 tablespoon lite soy sauce
6 ounces crabmeat (or immitation crabmeat)
1 8-ounce can water chestnuts, chopped
1/4 cup green onions, finely chopped
1/2 cup green bell pepper, finely chopped

Combine first 4 ingredients. Blend until fluffy. Add remaining ingredients and mix well. Cover and chill well. Garnish with paprika and parsley. Serve with a selection of fresh vegetables

yield, 2 cups
per serving information
18 calories per tablespoon

6.12 milligrams.cholesterol
.48 grams saturated fat
0.83 grams fat

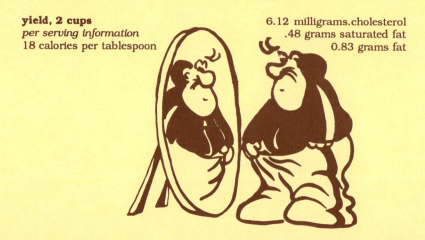

Vegetable Dip

1 cup low-fat cottage cheese
2 tablespoons skim milk
1 tablespoon green pepper, chopped
1 tablespoon green onion, chopped
1 tablespoon radish, chopped
1/2 teaspoon garlic salt

In a small bowl, beat cottage cheese and milk until creamy. Stir in remaining ingredients. Chill 2 to 3 hours. Serve with a selection of crisp fresh vegetables.

4 1/3-cup servings
per serving information
60 calories per 1/3 cup

3.5 milligrams cholesterol
.503 grams saturated fat
0.83 grams fat

Fruit Nibblers

1 cantaloupe
1 honeydew
4 to 6 pounds watermelon
2 to 3 oranges cut in half

Scoop balls from melons or cut into 1-inch cubes. Place 3 balls on each small bamboo skewer. Arrange orange halves on serving tray. Surround with fresh parsley. Insert skewers in orange halves. Serve orange juice in small bowl for dipping.

serving, 1 skewer
per serving information
30 calories

0.0 milligrams cholesterol
0.0 grams saturated fat
0.0 grams fat

230 Party Menus

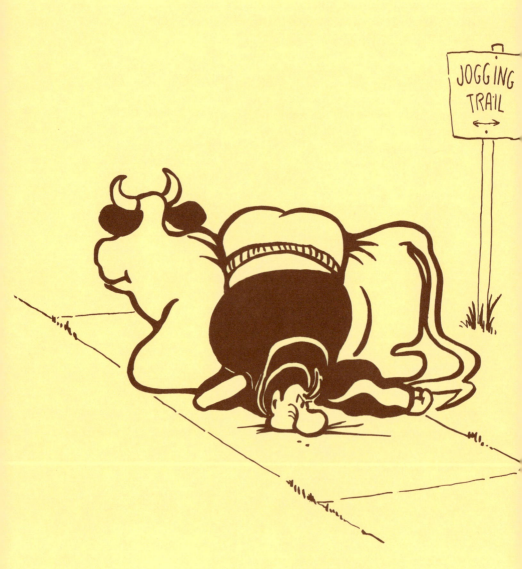

THE END

Recipe Index

Appetizers, non-beef
    Canapes, smoked salmon, 226
    Prosciutto, melon tidbits, 211
    Shrimp, deviled, 227
Barbeque
    Beef brisket, 129
    Filets with tarragon butter, 170
    North Carolina beef for a crowd, 217
Beef Salads
    Beef artichoke, 152
    Beef and asparagus, 74
    Beef and dill pickle, 82
    Beef, raspberry, and kiwi, 84
    California ground sirloin, 75
    Cold beef, with ginger dressing, 167
    Deluxe steak, 81
    Italian beef, 79
    Lime beef, 83
    Marinated beef, 78
    Pasta beef, 80
    Ross's beef, 77
    Spectacular cold beef, 184
    Tomato beef, 76
Brisket
    Beef barbeque, 129
    Beef, 126
    New England boiled dinner, 127
    North Carolina barbeque beef for a crowd, 217
Burgers
    Deluxe New Orleans, 107
    Louisiana, 107
    Ortega chili burgers, 106
    Super French burgers, 105
    Versatile burger, 104
Chateaubriand, 120

Cubed beef
    Curried sweet potato and, 143
    Spanish rice with, 141
Desserts
    Apples, poached, 165
    Bananas Foster, 159
    Bananas, sauteed, 195
    Cake,
        Mocha angel, 203
        Raspberry angel food delight, 206
    Cereal, sweet puffs, 220
    Cookies, meringue, 224
    Fresh fruit
        Compote, 200
        Nibblers, 229
        Marinated, 197
        Melons, polka dot, 157
        Mixed, 161, 163, 181, 189, 216
        Platter, 211, 224
        Strawberries with Grand Marnier, 169
    Grapefruit, baked, 177
    Mousse, amazing fake chocolate, 187
    Oatmeal, squares, 216
    Parfaits,
        Pineapple raspberry, 167
        Strawberry, 192
    Peach, summer delight, 185
    Sherbet,
        Lime, 155
        Raspberry, 179
        Strawberry, 175
    Souffle, orange, 172
    Sauce,
        Aloha, 163
        Raspberry for just about anything, 181

Dips
Cheese, 210
Cheesy fruit, 225
Chili, 218
Crab, 228
Horseradish, 221
Vegetable, 229
Fajitas, 136
Filet mignon, lemon garlic
accent with, 158
Filets
Barbeque with
tarragon butter, 170
Cheese and pepper
stuffing with, 168
Italian steaks, 190
Ground beef
"Camp-out" ground beef
soup, 90
Peppers, stuffed green, 144
Porcupines, 140
Shepherd's Pie, 146
Ground sirloin,
Sunday morning hash, 148
Texas skillet supper, 142
Tomatoes, stuffed with, 145
Kabobs
Broiled fruit, 153
Chinese beef, 226
Simple, 225
Vegetable, 218
Lasagne, low-calorie, 209
Marinade
Another great beef, 115
Burgundy, 116
Great beef, 114
Hawaiian, 116
Sesame lime, 117
Meat loaf, 196
Mexican, 176
Meatballs
Noodles and, 180
Oriental, 227
Wine with spaghetti
squash, 164

Pasta
Fettuccini with onion
wine sauce, 155
Noodles, green onion, 191
Parsleyed, 174
Pot Roast, deluxe, 194
Relish, fresh onion, 214
Ribs
Oriental garlic short, 131
Our favorite beef, 130
Roasts
Mustard barbequed
beef, 128
No-fail rib, 221
Secret marinated chuck, 213
Southwestern style beef, 125
Salad dressings
Caper, 184
Coleslaw, 179
Cottage cheese, 199
Creamy spring, 194, 219
Cucumber, 171
Dilly buttermilk, 165
Garlic yogurt, 157
Ginger, 167
Green salad, 175, 181
Horseradish, 152
Parsley, 161
Renn's red, 68
Spicy, 205
Vinaigrette, 211, 223
basic, 68
Salads
Artichoke, 169
Asparagus and grape, 179
Beet, fresh, 71
Caesar, 187
Cucumber, 181
Cucumber and
orange, 203
Cucumber lemon, 189
Sliced, 72
Green, 157, 161, 165, 171,
175, 194, 211, 219, 223
Green and white, 70

Hearts of palm, 70
Japanese, 69
Layered vegetable, 199
"Let's go camping" potato, 215
Orange kiwi with almonds,
176
Overnight vegetable, 196
Palm, hearts of with
asparagus, 71
Radish and strawberry, 197
San Francisco dinner, 69
Snow pea, 154
Three bean marinated, 215
Three color, 72
Tomatoes, beefsteak in spicy
dressing, 205
Salsa, fresh, 161
Sandwiches
Best beef you'll ever have, 110
Florentine beef pita
bread, 111
Low-calorie Sloppy Joes, 109
Open-faced beef, 112
Sauce
Dessert,
Aloha, 163
Raspberry for just about
anything, 181
Simple spaghetti, 138
Thick meat, 139
Yogurt dill, 196
Shepherd's Pie, 146
Soup
Albondigas, 202
Beef barley, 89
Beef vegetable for a crowd, 91
Beef vegetable rice, 88
Brandy beef, 87
Cajun black bean, 92
"Camp-out" ground beef, 90
Gazpacho, favorite, 210
Hearty lentil, 94
Oriental style hot and
sour, 86
Spicy red bean, 93

Steak
au poivre, 156
Hawaiian flank, 162
Italian, 190
London broil, 186
Marco Mexican tartar, 137
Marinated broiled, 188
Round, beef burgundy, 134
Sirloin strips, Hungarian
goulash, 147
Sirloin strips, skillet,
red wine, 135
Sirloin, dilly, 122-123
Sirloin, salsa marinated, 124
Sirloin, low-fat beef
stroganoff, 132
Sirloin, sweet and sour
grilled, 121
Southwestern grilled, 160
Stew, beer and beef, 133
Stir-fry
Beef with cashews, 97
Chinese beef and rice, 96
Orange beef, 101
Spicy beef and noodles, 102
Spicy broccoli beef, 100
Szechuan beef with
peanuts, 98
Tomato beef, 99
Tenderloin
Beef Dianne, 154
Mock, 204
Tips, teriyaki, 174
Vegetables
Asparagus,
with tart vinaigrette
dressing, 200
wrapped in prosciutto,
222
Beans,
Green herbed, 177
Tequila, 219
Broccoli,
marinated, 191
sweet and sour, 159

Chinese style, 163
Corn, summer, 171
Kabobs, vegetable, 218
Mushroom,
    stuffed caps, 228
    Italian stuffed, 156
    zucchini, 204
Onions, whole,
    roasted, 222
Peas, like fresh, 189
Potatoes,
    Baked beef stuffed, 178
    Low-calorie mashed, 195
    Mexican, 160
    Overbaked, 186
    Parsleyed, 168
    Stuffed baked, 205
    Twice baked, 157

Rice, wild Pilaf, 158
Rice, wild with fresh
    mushrooms, 188
Snow peas, sauteed, and
    cucumbers, 159
Spinach, broccoli and, 180
Spinach cheese
    casserole, 223
Tomato aspic, 170
Tomatoes,
    Beef stuffed, 145
    Beefsteak, in spicy
        dressing, 205
    Herb broiled, 190
Zucchini, Italian tomato,
    with parmesan
    cheese, 178
Zucchini, stuffed, 198

Beef Lover's Gifts
Handmade in Utah

Each item
♥ Carries designs of the Beef Lover's cow created for the series by Jerry Palen.

♥ Produced exclusively by expert seamstresses in Cedar City, Utah, of the finest quality materials and colors.

Sweat Shirt (cow jumping rope)
Sizes S M L XL
$39.95

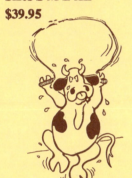

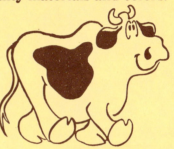

Chef's Apron
(walking cow)
poplin, full length
one size
$19.95

Kid's 2-piece Pajamas
(sitting cow)
Sizes   18 months to 4 $24.95
           6 to 8 $26.95

Kid's 2-piece Sweat Suits
(sitting cow)
Sizes 18 months to 4 $29.95
      6 to 8 $31.95

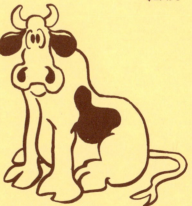

Creative Color Combinations available (all items)
(color must be specified on order form as W, P, Y, B, or T)
White with Black Cow   Pink with Purple Cow
Yellow with Turquoise Cow   Royal Blue with White Cow
Turquoise with Rust Cow

236　Party Menus

Order Form

			Price Each	Number Ordered	Total
The Beef Lover's Guide			$24.95		
Beef Gifts	size	color			
Kid's Pajamas					
Kid's sweats					
Adult sweats			$39.95		
Chef's aprons			$19.95		
Subtotal for gifts					
Postage & Handling (10% of total order-Min. $5)					
Texas Residents (add 6% sales tax)					
TOTAL ORDER					

Enclosed Check or Money Order (Pay to Portfolio Publishing Co.) ☐

☐ **Charge my**　　　**MasterCard** ☐　**VISA** ☐

Card number ———————————— Expiration Date ———

Signature ————————————————————

Name ————————————————————————

Address —————————————————————————

City ——————————————————————————

State ——————————— Zip ———————————————

Mail Orders to:
Portfolio Publishing Company, Inc.
PO Box 7802
The Woodlands, TX 77387
tel: 713/363-3577